SKI
DEEP

SKIN DEEP

NATURAL RECIPES
FOR HEALTHY SKIN AND HAIR

MARGARET DINSDALE

FIREFLY BOOKS

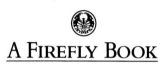

A FIREFLY BOOK

Cataloguing in Publication Data

Dinsdale, Margaret, 1953-
  Skin deep : natural recipes for healthy skin and hair

ISBN 0-921820-81-X

1. Skin - Care and hygiene. 2. Hair - Care and hygiene. 3. Herbal cosmetics. 4. Toilet preparations. I. Title.

RL87.D56 1998   646.7'2   C98-930787-5

Published in Canada in 1998 by
Firefly Books Ltd.
3680 Victoria Park Avenue
Willowdale, Ontario M2H 3KI

Published in the United States in 1998 by
Firefly Books (U.S.) Inc.
P.O. Box 1338, Ellicott Station
Buffalo, New York 14205

We acknowledge the financial support of the Government of Canada through the Book Publishing Industry Development Program for our publishing activities.

Design by
Linda J. Menyes

Photography by
Ernie Sparks

Illustrations by
Marta Scythes

Colour separations by
Hadwen Imaging Technologies
Ottawa, Ontario

Printed and bound in Canada by
Metropole Litho Inc.
St. Bruno de Montarville, Quebec

Thank you to the following companies for the loan of photo props:
Soap dish on cover, courtesy UMBRA, Scarborough, Ontario.
Brush, page 83, courtesy Soap Berry Shop, Kingston, Ontario.
Comb, page 84, courtesy Crabtree & Evelyn.

Dedicated to my two beautiful and cherished sons, Hamish and Alasdair

To the following, with gratitude: Patrick Lima and John Scanlan, for their love and friendship over the years; Laura Hubert, for giving me faith in myself and my abilities; my parents, Don and Beryl Dinsdale, for always supporting me in my various endeavours; Camden House staff Tracy Read, Linda Menyes, Susan Dickinson, Jane Good, Catherine DeLury and Mary Patton, for their infinite patience and sense of humour; and to all my friends, too numerous to name but who know who they are, each one precious and irreplaceable, who keep me laughing and singing.

CONTENTS

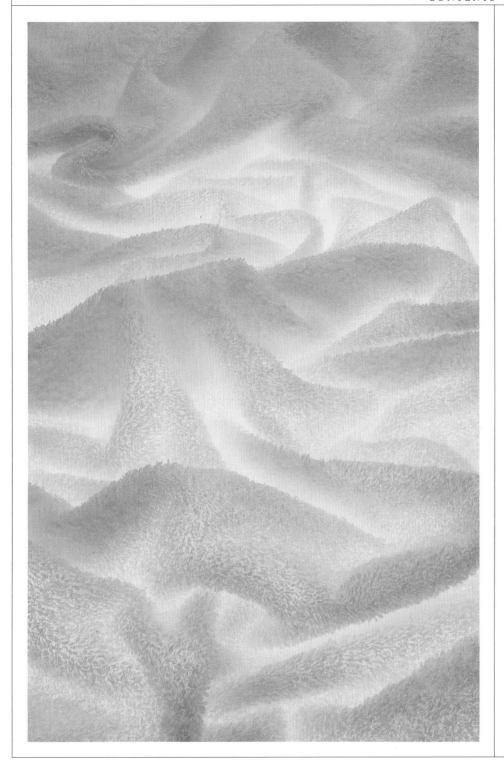

INTRODUCTION

At the end of a tiring day, I sometimes wander out into my garden, brush my hands against a mat of lemon thyme or Roman camomile and inhale deeply as the plant's essential oils are released into the air. There are few sensory experiences more delightful than the scent of aromatic herbs. My bed of mixed mints never fails to restore me; plantings of old, fragrant roses lead me to conjure up romantic fantasies; and clary sage, a tall biennial that has an extended blooming season, lends a particularly welcome fragrance to the garden. ❧ Scientific studies suggest that our sense of smell is the most powerful agent of memory stimula-

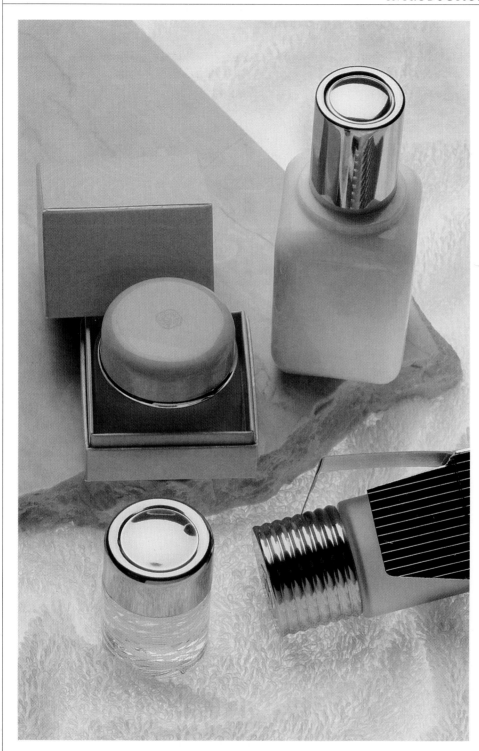

*Extravagant
displays, glossy
packaging and
high prices are
the norm in the
cosmetics
industry.*

tion. The associative power of scent has practical as well as imaginative implications: savvy real estate agents have been known to simmer a spice-laden stovetop potpourri to beguile prospective buyers into a cozy feeling of hominess. Poems, novels and essays have explored the profound human dependence upon smell. In *A Natural History of the Senses*, author Diane Ackerman observes: "We may not need to smell to survive, but without it, we feel lost and disconnected."

When we use natural substances, then, we affirm an important connection with our personal and collective roots. Every civilization in history has favoured certain aromatics that were incorporated into the cultural rituals of its society. Egyptians and Arabians used myrrh and frankincense for healing and embalming. Turks used the rose, the queen of aromatics, for skin care, scent and cooking. In India, patchouli and sandalwood are still two of the most popular essences. For North American natives, sweet grass is a sacred plant.

In the same way, our pervasive use of cosmetics and other skin preparations is a distinct echo of distant cultural practices. Archaeological evidence has proved that prehistoric peoples used pigments mixed with greasy substances to paint not only their dwellings but also their faces and bodies. As societies became more sophisticated, other materials were employed both for decoration—saffron and henna, for example—and for skin care—herbs such as thyme, rosemary and oregano and oils such as sweet almond, sesame and olive, to name a few. These common natural ingredients have been used all over the world.

At the same time, fashion has sometimes dictated styles that place effect ahead of health. In search of the alabaster skin tone that Elizabethan society deemed desirable, both men and women used face powder laced with poisonous white lead. Examples of the same surrender to trends are obvious during a walk down the streets of any 20th-century urban centre.

While most industrialized nations now have regulatory agencies that forbid the use of dangerous substances in cosmetic preparations, there is no agency that protects the consumer from the created appetite for goods. Whenever I stroll past the cosmetic counter in a department store or pharmacy, I experience a certain degree of despair, both at the amount of money that manufacturers are spending on the display counters themselves and at the enormous quantity of wasteful packaging that is used to persuade the consumer that these items are essential to their fashion—and therefore to their personal—success.

What bothers me more than this coercive prescription for acceptable grooming, however, is the lack of quality too often found in some of these product lines. I wince when I think of the fortunes that companies make selling little dabs of mineral oil, rendered animal wastes and synthetic fragrances cloaked in double-walled plastic containers and tucked into shiny little boxes. And all of this is inevitably accompanied by glossy brochures, manipulative sales pitches and astonishing prices.

My own way of wrestling with these pressures has been to explore the option of making some of these skin-care products myself. In my own home, I am able to oversee the quality of ingredients and to play with my own sensory responses, rather than simply passively inherit those created for me by a faceless committee of marketers. There have been immediate benefits: the wonderful sense of satisfaction one gets from self-sufficiency; the joy of creativity; the financial savings; and the opportunity to draw closer to the world of the garden, which is the original source of so many of these products.

As I was buying a cookbook the other day, I mentioned to the store manager that I was writing a "recipe" book myself, one that would teach people how to make their own natural skin-care items at home. Her assistant and another customer overheard our conversation and offered their comments.

"Oh, you mean putting yogurt on your skin," said one.

"Something like that," I replied.

"Yeah, like cucumbers on your eyes. All that old stuff," said the other.

The exchange made me think even more carefully about my intentions in writing this book. I knew what these women meant. I have seen lots in print about "natural skin care" that did indeed involve the ubiquitous cucumbers and yogurt. While these methods work, I, too, have hankered for something more.

How is this book different, and for whom is it written? Simply put, it is for consumers who are tired of spending so much on what seems so little, for people who suffer from skin sensitivities and allergies to the synthetic ingredients in manufactured skin-care products and for people who want to feel a little more in charge of what they rub onto their bod-

ies. There are straightforward recipes here that even the busiest person will have time to make. There are also more challenging recipes for those who are intrigued by the field. With a little time and effort and with relatively little cost, readers will be able to create a whole range of skin-care items, including cleansers, body splashes, facial toners and massage oils, that will be not only cheaper and more environmentally friendly but more effective as well.

SKIN TYPE

The New Encyclopaedia Britannica calls skin our "largest organ of identification and sexual attraction." In other words, our skin tells us—and others—just who we are. Every person's skin is unique, from its texture and scent to the troublesome characteristics it sometimes exhibits. For convenience' sake, however, I do refer to four general categories: normal, oily, dry, and sensitive or mature skin, and each recipe indicates the skin type for which it is best suited. Keep in mind that these descriptions are not ironclad, so when you are creating your own skin-care products, a little experimentation can be a good thing.

NORMAL SKIN

By normal skin, I do not mean perfect skin but, rather, skin that falls within a moderate range of health—skin that possesses good colour and texture, boasts few blemishes and is not particularly sensitive or allergic. People with normal skin may have occasional dry and/or oily areas on their face or body, but these are not problematic.

Even if your skin is normal, it still needs attention, especially to handle the artificial heating and cooling systems humans have devised to cope with the changing weather. Ill health, stress and pregnancy are just a few of the other factors that can affect your skin adversely.

OILY SKIN

Oily skin is generally characterized by large pores and an excess of secretions from the sebaceous glands. Blackheads and blemishes can sometimes accompany this skin type, as can dandruff. Although it may seem to be a contradiction, oily skin sometimes needs light moisturizing to hydrate it. Eating nutritional foods, drinking lots of water and using a mild cleanser morning and night can also help.

During hot, muggy weather, splash your face with water or toner, then blot it to reduce surface bacteria that can create new blemishes and to manage excess oil that can block pores. Preparations that contain a high amount of alcohol or another substance which tightens the pores can also block normal skin functions. Problems with oiliness or blemishes on other parts of the body, such as the upper back, will benefit from the same treatment as the face.

If you do have oily skin, take heart. People with this skin type seem to show their age a lot later than those with dry skin.

DRY SKIN

Skin that is chronically dry, regardless of the season, is referred to as dry skin. More dramatically, there may be flakiness, dandruff, tautness and cracking at the finger joints. Cleansing for dry skin should be very gentle. You do not want to strip away too much of the skin's natural secretions. Moisturizing with gentle,

emollient substances is essential, while misting the face during the day can help alleviate the drying effects of air conditioning or central heating.

Diet is also a vital consideration. Eat vegetables that contain vitamin C and beta carotene, and drink plenty of water. Make sure that you are getting enough oils in your diet.

SENSITIVE OR MATURE SKIN

As the skin ages, it thins, loses some of its elasticity and has a tendency to become drier. Fine lines appear, and recovery from trauma is slower. Although dryness seems to be a more common reaction, sensitivities can sometimes accompany either oily or dry skin. Such skin also reacts easily to chafing, irritation and some cosmetics, as well as developing allergic responses to clothing and other stimuli.

What each of these skin types needs is gentle cleansing and regenerative preparations that moisturize without blocking the pores. Any essential oils that are used should be mild and toning, and herbs with a good tannin or mucilage content are beneficial. Vitamins A, C and E and lots of water in the diet will help the skin to function normally.

USER-FRIENDLY SKIN CARE

Finally, a little advice on how best to use this book. Before attempting any of the recipes, please read the chapter "Methods & Equipment" thoroughly. There, you will find descriptions of the techniques necessary to make some of these items (it's not unlike learning how to make a sauce from a cookbook before you introduce it to a casserole). Of course, there are dozens of other recipes that require nothing more elaborate than a measuring cup, a bowl and a handful of herbs.

When you find a recipe that you would like to try, take note of the items you will need, then simply refer back to the chapter "Ingredients" for a listing of the plants, oils, essential oils, fruits and grains called for, as well as a detailed description of their benefits and properties. In no time at all, you could be indulging in a luxurious herbal bath of your own creation.

Give me an ounce of civet, good apothecary, to sweeten my imagination.
—William Shakespeare, *King Lear*

INGREDIENTS

Most of the ingredients for the recipes presented in this book are readily available from your neighbourhood grocery store, natural-food store or pharmacy; many can be grown in your backyard, gathered in the wild or even harvested from your lawn. ✺ This chapter is divided into three sections: The Kitchen, The Garden and The Pharmacy. In each, you will find an annotated list of ingredients that can be used in the creation of your own natural skin- and hair-care products. ✺ If you live in a community that is off the beaten track, don't despair. Mail-order houses in both Canada and the United States carry reliable lines of

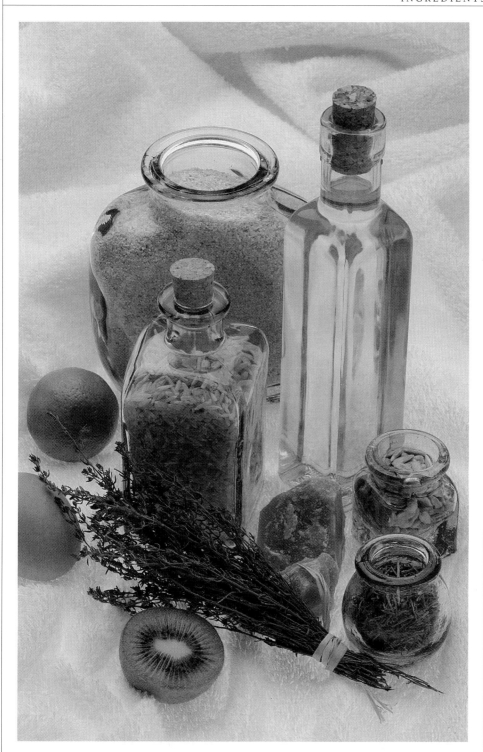

*Many of the
ingredients for
these recipes,
such as eggs,
oils, herbs
and fruit, are
as near at hand
as your pantry
or refrigerator.*

essential oils, quality herbs and other related items and will be happy to fill your
order. Also, many pharmacies will spe-
cial-order products at your request. For
more information about sources, turn
to page 104.

THE KITCHEN

In almost every kitchen, you will find a
number of ingredients that can be used
to create effective skin-care products.
Many everyday substances, such as milk
or yogurt, can be used either on their
own or in combination with other ingredients to prepare dozens of recipes in
this book. A list of some of these items
and their uses follows.

MILK

Milk is a very gentle cleanser that can be
used directly on the face or introduced
to the bath. For oily skin, use skim milk
or buttermilk; for dry skin, use milk with
a higher butterfat content.

Storage: refrigerator

YOGURT

Plain yogurt made from a bacterial cul-
ture, rather than gelatin, acts as a gentle
cleanser that is also soothing and cooling
for treating sunburns and minor skin
irritations. It can be used as a facial
cleanser or mask or for body packs and
scrubs. Blend half and half with water or
a herbal infusion, or use as is.

Storage: refrigerator

OILS

Oils are the base ingredient in most
moisturizers. They are also used in massage and for general skin care. Because of
their strength, essential oils (see page 29)
must be diluted before use, and the following carrier oils are most commonly
employed for this purpose. They can be
found in natural-food and grocery stores.

Apricot Kernel: A lovely light-textured oil
that is good for all skin types. Very mild
and soothing.

Avocado: Look for an avocado oil that is
dark green and aromatic; more refined
versions are lighter in colour and not as
rich. Excellent for very dry skin; only a
small amount is needed in a blend of
other oils. Contains protein and vitamins
A and B.

Coconut: See The Pharmacy.

Corn: Good middle-of-the-road oil for all
skin types. Look for golden colour and a
pleasant fragrance.

Flaxseed: Also known as linseed oil,
flaxseed oil is excellent as a hot poultice
for inflammatory skin disorders, such
as psoriasis and rashes, and is effective
for burns.

Grape-Seed: The most neutral vegetable
oil; high in polyunsaturates. Soothing
for sensitive, mature and infantile skin.
Fairly light texture; pale green in colour.

Jojoba: See The Pharmacy.

Olive: For skin care, use inexpensive
olive oil, rather than the expensive aromatic virgin brands. Emollient. Can be
gently heated and cooled without sub-
stantially altering its molecular structure.
To be used by those with dark complexions when sunbathing; also for dry skin.

Peanut: Very light. Good for oily skin or
for facial oils.

Rice Bran: Very light in texture and
colour. Gentle; good for very sensitive
and mature skin and for inflamed skin.

Sesame: It has been said that sesame oil
absorbs the sun's harmful ultraviolet
rays, which supposedly makes it an effective sunscreen. I wouldn't count on it
for protection, but the pressed oil is

wonderfully aromatic and emollient. Don't use the toasted Chinese variety unless you want to smell like a stir-fry.

Soya: A pale yellow oil, high in linoleic acid as well as oleic, stearic, palmitic and other acids. Soya oil is quickly absorbed by the skin.

Sunflower: Inexpensive, light and with little fragrance. Can be used to cut the richness of other oils, such as sweet almond. For all skin types.

Sweet Almond: A heavy emollient oil with a mild fragrance and a pale yellow colour. Pressed from almonds, this oil contains olein, glyceride and linoleic acid. Effective for dry skin and for diaper rash. For body massages, dilute half and half with a lighter oil, such as sunflower or apricot kernel. Do not confuse with bitter almond essential oil, which is used for flavouring.

Wheat Germ: Good wheat germ oil should be a rich golden colour and have a distinct slightly nutty aroma. Contains proteins, phosphorus and vitamin E. Only a small amount is needed in a blend of other oils. For all skin types.

Storage: refrigerator or dark, cool cupboard

GRAINS AND SEEDS

Almonds: Ground almonds are a gentle, effective cleanser for dry, sensitive skin on the body and face.

Barley: Soothing and emollient. Must be cooked, soaked or finely ground for use.

Bran: Use as is for gentle cleansing of the face and body or in body scrubs.

Cornmeal: For an abrasive action on the body, use the coarse meal. For gentle cleansing of the face, use a fine meal or flour.

Oatmeal: Very useful for gentle cleansing and for soothing red, sensitive skin. Use lightly ground rolled oats or oat flour.

Rice: Same as barley. Short-grain brown rice is the most emollient.

Sesame Seeds: Small, aromatic seeds that are rich in oils. Grind, with mortar and pestle, to use for cleansing dry or sensitive skin.

Sunflower Seeds: Same uses as almonds.

Storage: airtight containers away from light and heat

FRUIT AND VEGETABLES

A variety of fruit and vegetables are used in the recipes presented in this book— tomatoes, strawberries, bananas, pineapples, peaches, potatoes, carrots and cucumbers, among them. Incorporating these into natural skin-care recipes makes very practical use of overripe fruit and vegetables. You can also juice them, pour the liquid into ice-cube trays and store in the freezer until they can be introduced into toners, masks, and so on.

Storage: refrigerator or cool cupboard

AGAR

Extracted from seaweed, agar is an emollient thickener and a good substitute for gelatin. It helps emulsify liquids and is used in a variety of items, such as gels.

Storage: keep dry

EGGS

Eggs are plentiful and relatively inexpensive and provide two cosmetic ingredients in one package. The egg white is used as an astringent and binding agent for toning and tightening the pores. The egg yolk is high in lecithin and a number of fats and vitamins, including vitamin E, which makes it ideal for dry skin and hair treatments. The egg yolk can also be used in creams to aid in the emulsifying process, but remember that anything made with eggs should be either used immediately or stored in the refrigerator and used within a few days.

Storage: refrigerator

SALTS

Salts are useful for treating body toxins, psoriasis, eczema, muscular aches, and so on, and there are a number of kinds from which to choose.

Baking Soda: Also known as bicarbonate of soda, this inexpensive substance is a good bath additive and is excellent for cleaning teeth. Soothing and cleansing.

Kitchen, or Iodized, Salt: Its main component is sodium chloride blended with iodine as well as agents that keep it free-running. Its advantages are its low cost and availability.

Sea Salts: Several different sea salts are available. White sea salt is used in cooking. Unrefined sea salts, which are grey in colour and never dry out completely, are best suited for use in skin-care products because they contain many trace elements and minerals that are beneficial to the skin.

Storage: keep dry

THE GARDEN

Everywhere I've lived, I have had a garden that contained herbs, vegetables and flowers, all interplanted. The smallest yard I had measured about 15 feet square and had very poor soil. I didn't bother much with vegetables in that garden, since there wasn't a lot of sunlight either. Instead, I grew flowers, a narrow strip of Jerusalem artichokes to the side of the back porch, a plum tree, four varieties of hops, several mints and at least 20 other herbs, some of which were rather odd and ancient things.

If you don't have access to a garden, you can still grow several useful plants. Many herbs, such as parsley and basil, and some edible flowers take kindly to being grown in pots or under lights. If you don't have access to a plot or a pot, you can buy fresh herbs in many grocery stores and farmers' markets.

Other riches await you in your backyard. Your lawn can be a good source of skin-care raw materials (dandelion and plantain, for instance), provided it hasn't been sprayed with chemical herbicides and insecticides or had synthetic fertilizers spread over it.

Finally, there are many serviceable plants, such as St.-John's-wort and white pond lily, that can be gathered in the wild. Just be sure that you take them from an area which has not been exposed to chemical sprays. Also, the etiquette of plant gathering in the wild demands that you don't clean out a species from a given location. My rule of thumb is to take one out of every four plants in any one site. If you think of the entire world as your garden and treat it accordingly, you'll do all right. I've sometimes been spotted traipsing along abandoned railroad tracks gathering armfuls of sweet clover, a tall spike or two of mullein and huge roots of yellow dock and burdock.

If you intend to dry herbs, pick them at their peak. For above-ground plant materials, that means just as the plant is flowering or about to; for roots, it means in the late fall or early spring, when there is little or no above-ground growth. Dry them away from light or direct sources of heat, and store in airtight containers or brown paper bags. (Other methods of processing fresh herbs, such as tinctures and infused oils, are discussed in the chapter "Methods & Equipment.")

If you are unable to find a source for fresh herbs, quality dried herbs are fairly easy to obtain. Look for dried herbs that are stored in airtight containers away from direct light or sources of heat.

PLANT DIRECTORY

Please remember that the properties of the plants listed here are for cosmetic, or external, uses only. Although some of these plants are also listed under "Essential Oils" (page 29), the characteristics of an essential oil are, to some degree, different from those of the herb, and an essential oil is always far more potent than the herb itself.

For each entry, I have indicated which part(s) of the plant should be used, as well as the solvent (usually water or alcohol) that is necessary to release the desired properties of the plant. Before attempting any of the recipes in this book, read carefully the chapter "Methods & Equipment," in which the techniques for creating tinctures, infusions and infused oils from these herbs are described.

This information has been gleaned from a variety of sources. It is not intended to replace the qualified professional advice you should seek if you suffer from a chronic complaint. Before including any of these plants in a recipe, be absolutely sure that you have identified them correctly.

AGRIMONY

(*Agrimonia eupatoria*)
Part used: flowers, leaves
Solvent: boiling water
Mildly astringent; useful for stubborn and chronic skin rashes and for the healing of wounds.

ANGELICA

(*Angelica archangelica*)
Part used: root, leaves, seeds
Solvent: boiling water; alcohol
Though used mostly in cooking or for making liqueurs, angelica makes a very mild, aromatic wash for itchy skin and is also slightly deodorant. As a result, some people may experience an allergenic reaction to it.

ARNICA

(*Arnica montana*)
Part used: flower heads, root
Solvent: boiling water; alcohol; oil
As an infused oil or a tincture, arnica is useful in small quantities for treating bruises, sprains, pain and shock.

BALM OF GILEAD

(*Populus* spp)
Part used: buds
Solvent: boiling water; alcohol; oil
Several varieties of North American poplar yield balsamic and resinous buds (more commonly known as poplar buds) that are high in salicylic acid and oleoresins. When infused in oil or as a tincture and rubbed onto the skin, balm of Gilead is warming; excellent for lessening the pain of arthritic conditions and bruises.

BASIL

(*Ocimum basilicum*)
Part used: leaves
Solvent: water
The popular pesto ingredient has many cosmetic uses as well. As a compress, it helps to relieve headaches and anxiety. It is also refreshing as a body splash or bath additive. The macerated leaves are a good poultice for insect stings.

BAY LAUREL
(*Laurus nobilis*)
Part used: leaves, berries
Solvent: water
The leaves of this plant are the bay leaves we use in cooking. Helpful in relieving pain of rheumatism as well as sprains and bruises; also used as an antiseptic. Bay laurel is an effective rinse or hair dressing for oily scalps or dandruff.

BIRCH
(*Betula pendula*)
Part used: leaves, bark
Solvent: alcohol; boiling water
Young leaves are mildly antiseptic. Toss in the bath to treat rheumatism and skin conditions such as eczema. The bark contains phenol and sulphur compounds, making it antiparasitic but also mildly irritating. Birch tar oil has the same properties and is effective for treating dry-scalp conditions.

BLADDER WRACK
(*Fucus vesiculosus*)
Part used: whole plant
Solvent: water; alcohol
If gathered from unpolluted waters, this seaweed is an excellent nutritive food, but it is also useful for skin care. Scientific studies have shown that it binds to radioactive strontium and draws it from the body. As a cold poultice, it is said to be useful for treating bruises and swollen glands. It also contains algin, which is soothing to the skin, and most of the vitamin complexes, as well as many trace elements and minerals. Use in facial masks, body packs and the bath.

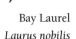

Bay Laurel
Laurus nobilis

BORAGE
(*Borago officinalis*)
Part used: flowers, leaves
Solvent: water
Contains mucilage, saponins and tannins. Soothing and cooling, borage is used to treat skin inflammations.

BURDOCK
(*Arctium lappa*)
Part used: root, leaves, seeds (burs)
Solvent: alcohol (root, burs); boiling water (root, leaves); oil (burs)
A tincture or an infusion of the root is an effective skin cleanser. Infused in oil or alcohol, the burs can be used for psoriasis, eczema and dry, scaly skin. The bruised or crushed leaves can be applied as a cooling poultice for fever or bruises.

CALENDULA
(*Calendula officinalis*)
Part used: flowers
Solvent: water; alcohol; oil
The English call this flower marigold, but don't confuse it with the common ornamental plant North Americans call marigold. Calendula is excellent for treating a variety of inflammations and rashes of the skin. It is also a recommended herb in a rinse for fair hair.

CAMOMILE, GERMAN
(*Matricaria chamomilla*)
Part used: flowers
Solvent: water; alcohol; oil
This common aromatic herb-tea plant is also a remedy for a long list of skin complaints, such as bruises and dry or sensitive skin. As an infused oil, it is useful for those same conditions as well as earache. Put a warmed drop in the ear, and gently place a bit of cotton batting over it. It is also a recommended herb in a rinse for fair hair. (See "Hair Care" chapter.)

CAMOMILE, ROMAN
(*Anthemis nobile*)
Part used: flowers, leaves
Solvent: water; alcohol; oil
Wonderfully aromatic, Roman camomile can be used as a compress for treating wounds, burns and swellings and is also good for dry, sensitive or mature skin. As an infused oil, it can be used to treat children's skin.

CHICKWEED
(*Stellaria media*)
Part used: stems, leaves
Solvent: water; alcohol
Containing mineral salts and saponins, this humble garden weed is most effective when it is fresh. Use as a cooling poultice or as an ointment for arthritis, scabs, boils, haemorrhoids and other skin conditions. It is also effective when used in a wash for greasy skin. Toss some in your salad as a spring tonic.

CLARY SAGE
(*Salvia sclarea*)
Part used: leaves, flowers, seeds
Solvent: water; alcohol
Clary sage seeds, soaked in water, yield a good quantity of mucilage, which can in turn be used as an ingredient in an eyewash. The aromatic flowers produce an essential oil that is highly touted as an aid for menstrual cramps. The leaves and flowers are astringent, cooling and soothing for general skin care.

CLEAVERS
(*Galium aparine*)
Part used: whole plant
Solvent: cold water
Also known as goosegrass, this rough little plant is very cooling and can help treat psoriasis, eczema and sunburn. Best used as a wash or an ointment.

CLOVER, RED
(*Trifolium pratense*)
Part used: flower heads
Solvent: water; alcohol
As a poultice or wash, red clover is effective in treating burns, sores and chronic skin ailments.

CLOVER, SWEET
(*Melilotus alba*)
Part used: flowers, leaves
Solvent: water; alcohol
Also known as melilot, this tall, sweetly scented field escapee is a common sight in midsummer. As a wash, a tincture or an ointment, it heals a variety of skin complaints that require a mild antibacterial agent. Sachets of the dried flowering plant add a sweet meadow scent to the linen cupboard.

CLOVER, YELLOW SWEET
(*Melilotus officinalis*)
Same characteristics and uses as sweet clover.

COMFREY
(*Symphytum officinale*)
Part used: leaves, root
Solvent: water; oil
With comfrey's very high content of mucilage and allantoin, an infusion or infused oil treats dry-skin conditions as well as bruises and minor wounds. A poultice helps severe bruising. Strengthens and softens the skin.

CORNFLOWER
(*Centaurea cyanus*)
Part used: flowers
Solvent: water

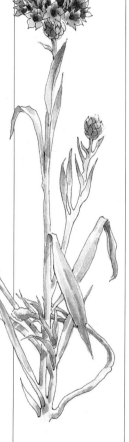

Cornflower
*Centaurea
cyanus*

A mild tonic and astringent. Useful as an ingredient in both an eyewash and a rinse for grey or white hair.

COWSLIP
(*Primula veris*)
Part used: flowers, leaves
Solvent: water
Made into an ointment, especially with flaxseed or coconut oil, cowslip can be used to treat a variety of burns. For general skin care, it softens and nourishes the skin.

DANDELION
(*Taraxacum officinale*)
Part used: root
Solvent: boiling water; alcohol
A tincture made from the root is useful in treating acne and skin eruptions.

DOCK, YELLOW OR CURLED
(*Rumex crispus*)
Part used: root
Solvent: water; alcohol
Tonic and astringent, a tincture made from the root is useful in treating acne and hives. It is also thought to aid in the control of ringworm and scabies.

ECHINACEA
(*Echinacea angustifolia*)
Part used: root
Solvent: alcohol; boiling water
As a wash or tincture, this is an effective remedy for boils, acne and abscesses.

ELDER
(*Sambucus canadensis*)
Part used: leaves, flowers
Solvent: water; alcohol (flowers)
As an ointment, the leaves are useful for treating sore joints, bruises and burns. (The leaves can be combined with camomile for this purpose.) Made into a water, a tincture, an oil or an ointment, the flowers soften the skin.

EUCALYPTUS
(*Eucalyptus globulus*)
Part used: leaves
Solvent: alcohol; water
Highly antiseptic yet mild in its action on the skin, this herb is useful as a bath additive. The diluted essential oil, either added to the bath or included in a massage oil, is good for colds, headaches, sinus congestion, muscular aches and pains, joint aches and fevers.

EVENING PRIMROSE
(*Oenothera biennis*)
Part used: plant (best when fresh), seeds
Solvent: water
The fresh plant makes an effective wash for minor wounds and skin eruptions. The seed oil, which you must buy rather than make, is a useful addition to skin treatments for dry or mature skin.

EYEBRIGHT
(*Euphrasia officinalis*)
Part used: flowers, leaves
Solvent: boiling water
High in tannins, this plant is widely used as an eyewash for conjunctivitis and other problems. It is also used for healing wounds.

FENNEL
(*Foeniculum vulgare*)
Part used: seeds
Solvent: boiling water; alcohol
Disinfectant and anti-inflammatory, fennel can be used as a detoxifying bath additive and as an eyewash for puffy eyes.

GERANIUM, SCENTED
(*Pelargonium* spp)
Part used: leaves
Solvent: water; alcohol
The most popular of this species, the rose geranium (*P. graveolens*) is a pleasantly scented houseplant. Along with the

many other varieties of scented geraniums, such as lemon, lime and apple, it is a soothing, balancing agent for all skin types. Good for treating scar tissue, inflammation, eczema, shingles and acne. Cooling compress for engorged breasts.

GOLDENROD
(*Solidago canadensis*)

Part used: leaves, flowers

Solvent: water

This much-maligned common weed was used by native peoples as a wash for treating wounds and ulcers. Mildly astringent.

GROUND IVY
(*Glechoma hederacea*)

Part used: flowers, leaves

Solvent: water; oil

Also known as gill-over-the-ground and ale hoof, ground ivy can be used as a wash or an infused oil for sluggish circulation and bruises. It is also suited for any preparation for the legs. Helps heal scabs and itchy rashes.

HEARTSEASE
(*Viola tricolor*)

Part used: flowers, leaves

Solvent: water

Commonly known as Johnny-jump-up, this herb is effective for chronic skin complaints. The salicylic acid content helps treat rheumatism. Heartsease is mildly stimulating, making it useful for sluggish circulation and fevers.

HORSE CHESTNUT
(*Aesculus hippocastanum*)

Part used: pulverized seeds

Solvent: boiling water; alcohol

Anti-inflammatory, antispasmodic. Use as a bath additive or a rub to help strengthen arteries and veins and relieve haemorrhoids. Useful for fluid retention.

HORSETAIL
(*Equisetum arvense*)

Part used: stems

Solvent: boiling water; oil

Astringent. High in silicic acid, horsetail aids the healing of wounds. As an infusion or infused oil, it can help strengthen hair shafts and nails.

HYSSOP
(*Hyssopus officinalis*)

Part used: flowers, leaves

Solvent: water; alcohol

High in tannins. Used as a wash, it is good for minor cuts, rheumatism and bruises and also acts as a mild circulation stimulant.

JUNIPER
(*Juniperus communis*)

Part used: berries, needles

Solvent: boiling water; alcohol

Juniper is warming and is widely used in Germany and Scandinavia as an antiseptic and for treating minor wounds, rheumatism, pulled muscles and bruises. Also diuretic, it is helpful with oily skin, eczema and fluid retention.

KELP
(*Alaria esculenta*)

See Bladder Wrack.

LADY'S MANTLE
(*Alchemilla vulgaris*)

Part used: leaves

Solvent: water

Astringent and styptic because of its tannin content, lady's mantle is good for toning skin and for wounds and bruises.

Cowslip
Primula veris

LAVENDER

(*Lavandula angustifolia* or *L. officinalis*)

Part used: flowers

Solvent: water; oil; alcohol

Mildly scented yet powerfully antiseptic, this is a most-maligned herb, being commonly sold inundated with cloyingly sweet artificial fragrances. Real lavender has a clean, spiky scent. It is soothing, deodorant and balancing for both dry and oily skins. Particularly useful in treating acne, burns and scalds, lavender can also be used to help soothe nervous conditions. As an added benefit, it keeps moths away from clothes.

LEMON BALM

(*Melissa officinalis*)

Part used: flowers, leaves

Solvent: water

A popular herb-tea component, this delicate plant is useful as a compress for headaches and nervousness and is soothing to the skin. Used in anti-rheumatic ointments and baths.

LEMON VERBENA

(*Aloysia triphylla*)

Part used: leaves

Solvent: water

Its delightful scent is enough reason to use lemon verbena, but it is also antispasmodic and useful for indigestion as well as treating acne.

LICORICE

(*Glycyrrhiza glabra*)

Part used: root

Solvent: water

This common flavouring agent makes a pleasant ointment or poultice for treating redness of the skin, eczema and psoriasis.

LINDEN

(*Tilia cordata*)

Part used: flowering bracts, leaves

Solvent: boiling water

The sweet-smelling flowers of the linden tree, known as lime tree in Europe, are useful in baths for relieving chills and flu symptoms. As a poultice, the leaves and flowers are effective for treating boils and painful swellings. Mildly diuretic and refreshing for general skin care.

LOVAGE

(*Ligusticum scoticum*)

Part used: root

Solvent: boiling water

Smelling strongly of celery, the leaves are used as a culinary flavouring. As a bath additive, the root is mildly diuretic, aromatic and deodorant.

MALLOW, COMMON

(*Malva sylvestris*)

Part used: leaves, flowers

Solvent: water; oil

A common lawn weed in temperate countries, mallow is soothing and anti-inflammatory. High in mucilage. Good for dry skin and as a poultice for sores and boils.

MARJORAM

(*Origanum majorana*)

Part used: flowers, leaves

Solvent: water; oil

A very soothing, aromatic herb used as an infused oil for the treatment of bruises, chills, flu, sinus congestion, muscular aches and coughs. The herb itself pleasantly scents the bath and is mildly antiseptic and calming.

MARSHMALLOW

(*Althaea officinalis*)

Part used: leaves, flowers, dried root

Solvent: water; oil

Very emollient and contains 10 percent mucilage; soothing as well. Relieves inflammation and dry-skin conditions.

NETTLE, STINGING
(*Urtica dioica*)
Part used: leaves
Solvent: boiling water
The chlorophyll found in the nettle leaves makes it a useful deodorant. It is astringent and stimulating, which is toning for the skin, and helps dandruff and oily scalps.

ORRISROOT
(*Iris florentina*)
Part used: dried root
Solvent: water; alcohol
The powdered or chopped dried root of this iris smells slightly of violet. It is often used as a fixative in potpourris and is also aromatic, mildly diuretic and deodorant for cosmetic uses.

PARSLEY
(*Petroselinum crispum*)
Part used: leaves, root, seeds
Solvent: water; oil; alcohol
Mildly diuretic, parsley leaves are useful as a wash and a bath additive. The infused oil or a tincture of the seeds is effective in treating acne.

PEPPERMINT
(*Mentha piperita*)
Part used: leaves
Solvent: water
This common toothpaste additive can also be used in the bath to treat headaches, sinus congestion, nausea, overheating and chills. It is also useful as a cooling agent in hot weather and for soothing skin rashes. (This applies to most mints, except pennyroyal.) Other mints that are useful for skin care are apple mint (*M. suaveolens*), curly mint (*M. spicata crispata*), ginger mint (*M. gentilis aureo-variegata*), orange mint (*M. citrata*) and spearmint (*M. spicata*).

PLANTAIN
(*Plantago major*)
Part used: leaves, seeds
Solvent: water; oil
As a wash or an infused oil, plantain is very emollient and is therefore good for dry-skin conditions. This common lawn weed is also mildly astringent and can be used on minor wounds.

ROSE
(*Rosa* spp)
Part used: petals, buds, hips
Solvent: water, alcohol (petals, buds, hips); oil (petals, buds)
Rose petals and buds are an aromatic bath additive, while rose water is very soothing for the eyes and good for toning inflamed or mature skin. Roses are a powerful antiseptic, hence their wonderful fragrance is a little surprising. The hips, when boiled slightly, strained and added to bathwater or lotion, soften the skin.

ROSEMARY
(*Rosmarinus officinalis*)
Part used: leaves
Solvent: water; alcohol; oil
Very antiseptic, rosemary is a stimulating, aromatic herb. Used in massage oils, bath additives and creams for sluggish circulation, muscle strains and joint pains. It is a tonic for oily skin and is used as a rinse for dark hair.

Rose Hips
Rosa spp

SAGE, COMMON
(*Salvia officinalis*)
Part used: leaves
Solvent: boiling water; alcohol
This common garden and kitchen herb is antiseptic, antifungal, anti-inflammatory and astringent. It is useful for toning the skin without drying it.

ST.-JOHN'S-WORT
(*Hypericum perforatum*)
Part used: flowers, leaves
Solvent: boiling water; alcohol; oil
An oil or a diluted tincture of this plant can be used wherever there is bruising, burns, mild wounds or haemorrhoids. Use sparingly.

SAVORY
(*Satureja hortensis; S. montana*)
Part used: flowers, leaves
Solvent: water; alcohol
Both summer and winter savory are similar to oregano and thyme in that they are highly antiseptic, making them effective as a refreshing gargle and as a treatment for minor scrapes and foot problems, such as athlete's foot. Can be substituted for thyme in skin-care recipes.

SELF-HEAL
(*Prunella vulgaris*)
Part used: flowers, leaves
Solvent: water
Also known as allheal and heal-all, this weed has a high tannin content that makes it useful as a wash for skin irritations, inflammation and minor wounds.

SILVERWEED
(*Potentilla anserina*)
See Tormentil.

SOAPWORT
(*Saponaria officinalis*)
Part used: root, leaves
Solvent: boiling water
High in saponins, the fresh leaves, infused, are a mild soap substitute. The root, as a bath additive or a wash, is helpful for psoriasis, eczema and acne.

SOUTHERNWOOD
(*Artemisia abrotanum*)
Part used: leaves
Solvent: water; oil
Used as a skin tonic for stimulating the circulation and toning oily skin.

SPEARMINT
(*Mentha spicata*)
See Peppermint.

SPEEDWELL
(*Veronica officinalis*)
Part used: flowers, leaves
Solvent: water; alcohol
This common roadside weed with its pale blue flowers has tannins and resins that make it a mild healing wash or bath additive for a wide range of skin complaints.

STRAWBERRY
(*Fragaria vesca*)
Part used: fruit, leaves
Solvent: boiling water (leaves)
The fruit is mildly acid, which makes it an effective skin cleanser. High in tannin, the leaves can be used to tone and soothe the skin.

THYME, GARDEN
(*Thymus vulgaris*)

THYME, WILD
(*Thymus serpyllum*)
Part used: leaves, flowers
Solvent: boiling water; alcohol
Thyme is highly antiseptic and germicidal. Since it has a stimulating effect, it is useful as a bath additive and for treating wounds and rheumatism. It is also used for foot soaks and as a treatment for acne and dandruff.

TORMENTIL
(*Potentilla erecta*)
Part used: root
Solvent: water; white vinegar
This wild plant yields a high amount of tannin, which is astringent, toning and anti-inflammatory. It is useful as a wash for treating burns, sunburn, haemorrhoids and abrasions.

VALERIAN
(*Valeriana officinalis*)
Part used: dried root
Solvent: water; alcohol
Use sparingly as a sedative bath additive.

VERVAIN
(*Verbena officinalis*)
Part used: flowers, leaves
Solvent: water
This herb contains mucilage, tannins and saponins, which aid in the treatment of wounds and chronic skin complaints.

VIOLET, SWEET
(*Viola odorata*)
Part used: whole plant
Solvent: boiling water; oil
As an infused oil, an ointment or a bath additive, this sweet-smelling flowering herb is mildly diuretic, cooling and deodorant. It was once used in the treatment of rheumatism, cancerous tumours and sore throats.

WHITE POND LILY
(*Nymphaea odorata*)
Part used: root
Solvent: water; alcohol
Indigenous peoples used this root to treat painful swellings, boils and ulcers. A wash made with white pond lily root and a bit of lemon juice is toning and restorative for the skin. A wash without lemon juice soothes tender skin, especially around the eyes.

WILD MARJORAM,
OR WILD OREGANO
(*Origanum vulgare*)
See Marjoram.

YARROW
(*Achillea millefolium*)
Part used: leaves, flowers
Solvent: water; alcohol; oil
Useful for oily skin and sluggish circulation. Also as a wash for minor wounds, haemorrhoids, rashes and abrasions. Use sparingly.

THE PHARMACY

Modern pharmacies feature vast aisles of hair-, skin- and face-care products. But if you look carefully, there is usually a section devoted to "old-time" items, such as rose water, borax, Epsom salts and eucalyptus essential oil, among others. There are also plain soaps, such as glycerin and olive oil (Castile), which are used in this book. If you don't see an ingredient that you want, ask the pharmacist. If it's available, most pharmacists will be happy to order it for you.

Many natural-food stores carry similar items, as well as an assortment of essential oils, plant tinctures and a variety of other products.

ALOE VERA GEL
Pure aloe vera gel is a thin, slightly brownish liquid. It is often preserved with citric acid. Some manufacturers add a seaweed thickener, usually carrageenan. To use fresh, cut a piece of the leaf from the plant and squeeze the gel directly onto the skin.

ASCORBIC ACID
More commonly known as vitamin C, this white powder is a good antioxidant and preservative for creams and lotions.

BEESWAX

Buy pure unbleached beeswax that is unadulterated with paraffin, which gives it gloss and a slightly slippery feeling. The beeswax you use should be free of foreign particles and have a golden brownish colour and a sweet fragrance. It is used in making creams and ointments. (A convenient way to handle beeswax: If you buy it in a large block, heat until it melts, then pour into an ice-cube tray. Each portion will measure approximately ⅛ cup, or 25 mL.)

BENZOIN

A resinous, aromatic tree gum that is frequently sold as a tincture, benzoin (*Styrax benzoin*) has a pleasant fragrance and is often used as a binding agent in facial toners and moisturizing lotions. It is antiseptic and preservative.

BORAX

Not to be confused with boric acid, borax (hydrated sodium borate) is a naturally occurring mild alkaline substance, sold as a powder, that softens water and is used in a wide variety of cosmetic preparations. Only a small quantity is needed.

CASTILE SOAP

An unscented, slightly acid olive oil soap that may be white, cream or green in colour. Made from olive oil and sodium hydroxide, it is also known as Marseilles soap and Greek olive oil soap. Can be grated and blended with water to make shampoo or liquid soap.

CASTOR OIL

A very rich, smooth oil used commercially in the manufacture of lipstick. Contains fatty acids and glycerin. When blended with other oils, it is an excellent treatment for very dry skin. Because it dries quickly upon exposure to air, it is useful in hair and nail treatments.

CITRIC ACID

An acid obtained by the fermentation of citrus fruit sugars, citric acid is a preservative and a foam inhibitor in cosmetics. Highly astringent, it is useful for toning the skin.

COCONUT OIL

A very fatty oil that is solid at room temperature, although it melts easily at slightly higher temperatures. It absorbs quickly and makes a light-textured cream or ointment.

EPSOM SALTS

A mild alkaline salt that disperses easily in water, this is excellent in the bath for soothing skin inflammations and muscular aches.

FLOWER WATERS

Some of the varieties available are rosemary, lavender, camomile, rose and orange. Some are for external use only; check the label to determine whether the flower water can be ingested.

FULLER'S EARTH

Also known as white clay, this powder is a useful additive to body powders and makes an excellent mask or body pack for drawing impurities from the skin. Other kinds, such as green clay, contain a different mineral composition but have the same general effect.

GLYCERIN

A by-product of the soap industry, this mildly alkaline liquid is a useful humectant for moisturizing the skin. It can be used on its own, mixed with rose water or added to creams and lotions. It may be animal- or vegetable-based, depending on whether tallow was used in the original process.

JOJOBA OIL

Pure jojoba oil is thick and pale yellow in colour; it is actually a liquid wax that dries rapidly upon exposure to air. Most commercial cosmetic jojoba oils are blends of jojoba and another oil, usually mineral.

LANOLIN

Lanolin is the yellowish fat that is gleaned from sheep wool. It is useful in treating very dry skin conditions and in the manufacture of creams. Look for water-free anhydrous lanolin.

LECITHIN

Soya lecithin is sold in capsules or as bulk liquid. (Lecithin is found in egg yolk, soya and brains.) An emulsifier and spreading agent, it is also an antioxidant and emollient that blends well with oil. Do not use the granules for cosmetics.

MYRRH TINCTURE

A resinous tree gum infused in alcohol, tincture of myrrh can be used in aqueous solutions to treat mouth infections and to tone the skin.

ORANGE FLOWER WATER

Whether made from the expensive pure neroli essential oil (orange blossoms) or the less costly petitgrain essential oil (orange-blossom leaves), this is a pleasantly scented, toning and soothing water for all skin types. It is also used in baking and in Middle Eastern cooking.

ROSE WATER

Traditionally, this was the water left after steam distillation of pure rose essential oil. Now, it is commonly made of a solution of pure rose essential oil distilled with water. Very soothing and toning for the eyes, dry or inflamed skin and mature skin. Rose water is also used in Middle Eastern and Indian cooking.

RUBBING ALCOHOL

This inedible liquid, also known as isopropyl alcohol, has additives that render it unfit for internal consumption, and its overpowering smell makes it unsuitable for most cosmetic uses. On its own or infused with herbs or essential oils, however, it is an effective rub for fevers, bedsores and strained muscles. Remember that anything containing rubbing alcohol should always be labelled with a skull and crossbones or other notation to indicate that it is poisonous.

VITAMIN E

Vitamin E is usually sold in capsules and is occasionally available in liquid form in bulk quantities. Externally used, it not only is an antioxidant for creams and oils but is also very healing for burns, scrapes and haemorrhoids.

WITCH HAZEL

Highly astringent, witch hazel is an excellent toner for oily, blemished skin and is also effective for treating bruises and haemorrhoids. Because of its strength, it should be used sparingly.

ESSENTIAL OILS

One of the most misunderstood items on the market, essential oils are the pure, undiluted and, for the most part, steam-distilled volatile oils from certain herbs, flowers and trees. Most have antiseptic, germicidal and preservative characteristics. Pure essential oils should not be used directly on the skin in their uncut state (with the sole exception of lavender), because undiluted essential oils can cause severe irritation and may even be toxic. A quick test to determine whether an essential oil is uncut is to put a *tiny* drop on the back of your hand and stroke a finger across it several times. It should evaporate quickly. Sandalwood, patchouli, cedar wood and several other oils are naturally thick and so will not conform to this test, but most oils will.

Unfortunately, there are imposters on the market. While there are no foolproof tricks to avoid buying a diluted oil, here are a few guidelines. Remember that most fruits do not produce an essential oil, so in all likelihood, products named strawberry, blueberry or apple essential oil are *not* essential oils. If the merchant suggests that you can apply them to your skin, you've probably stumbled onto a hybrid, rather than the real thing.

Likewise, there are perfume oils sold as essential oils that are actually a mixture of synthetic and natural fragrance compounds and do not possess therapeutic qualities. They should be used only for their fragrance, while potpourri refresher oils should *never* be used on the skin or in the bath. Even if they claim to be made of real essential oils, most potpourri refreshers contain spice oils or preservatives that render them totally unsuitable for skin care.

Finally, pure essential oils vary widely in price, from inexpensive citrus oils to the more expensive sandalwood, pure rose and pure jasmine essential oils. Check the labels carefully. The more expensive essential oils, such as pure neroli and Roman camomile, are sometimes sold in a dilution of 10 percent in sweet almond oil, which is perfectly acceptable as long as you know the percentage of the dilution when you use the essential oil in a recipe.

Essential oils should be stored in brown glass bottles, away from direct light. Handle with care. Some oils will melt plastic in their uncut state. Wash thoroughly with soap and water if any uncut essential oil spills on your skin.

A NOTE ON WORKING WITH ESSENTIAL OILS

A herb and its essential oil can have very different properties and potencies. Do *not* use an essential oil as a direct substitute for a herb in any of the recipes in this book unless instructed to do so. And remember, essential oils should *never* be taken internally.

"Recommended dilution" refers to the total quantity of an oil called for in a massage oil, cream, and so forth. A 2 percent dilution, for example, would mean the addition of 40 drops pure essential oil to ½ cup (125 mL) carrier oil. If you wish to combine two essential oils, simply halve the dilution of each in order to avoid creating an overpowering effect. If using three, reduce the dilution of each by a third, and so on.

AROMATHERAPY-STRENGTH MASSAGE OR BATH OIL

Recommended dilution: 2% to 5%
This dilution can be used either on selected areas of the body or in quantities of 1 to 2 tsp. (5-10 mL) for the bath.

To ¼ cup (50 mL) carrier oil, such as sweet almond or grape-seed, add 20 to 50 drops essential oil and the contents of ½ capsule of vitamin E. Blend well, bottle, and label.

TOTAL BODY MASSAGE OIL

Recommended dilution: ½% to 2%
In ¼ cup (50 mL) carrier oil, such as sweet almond or grape-seed, add 5 to 20 drops essential oil and the contents of 1 capsule of vitamin E. Blend well, bottle, and label.

FOR THE BATH

Add 2 to 8 drops essential oil to the bathwater, and briskly agitate water before entering. Essential oils introduced into the bath are even more effective if they are mixed first with a mild shampoo or liquid soap.

Please Note: The following essential oils should *not* be used in the bath, because they are too harsh and will irritate the skin as well as the mucous membranes: birch tar, bitter almond, cade, camphor, cedar leaf, cedar wood, cinnamon, citronella, cloves, hawthorn, hyssop, mother-of-thyme, myrrh, nettle, nutmeg, origanum, patchouli, pennyroyal, red thyme, sassafras, savory, turpentine, white thyme or wintergreen.

INHALATIONS

Add 2 to 4 drops essential oil to a bowl of hot water. Make a tent over the bowl with a towel, and inhale the steam for several minutes. Recommended essential oils for sinus and respiratory problems are: eucalyptus, frankincense, black pepper, basil, peppermint and balsam fir.

LOTIONS

Mix 2 to 5 drops essential oil in a little grain alcohol or vodka. Add ¼ cup (50 mL) distilled water. Shake well before using. For dry skin, add ½ tsp. (2 mL) glycerin.

SOME COMMON ESSENTIAL OILS

Not a complete reference, this list includes readily available essential oils.

BALSAM FIR
(*Abies balsamea*)
Recommended dilution: 1% to 5%
Balsam fir essential oil is obtained by steam-distilling the resin that is collected by tapping the trees. It is mild and gently warming and so lends itself to treating sore muscles, colds and flu.

BASIL
(*Ocimum* spp)
Recommended dilution: 1% to 3%
Spicy and aromatic, basil is excellent for headaches, migraines, sinus infections, stress and hay fever. It is warming and antiseptic. Add it to massage or bath oils to soothe and warm. In a massage oil, rub into the temples, neck and shoulders when tension or a headache is ruining your day. Put a drop or two of basil essential oil in a bowl of hot water for an effective sinus inhalation.

BERGAMOT ORANGE
(*Citrus aurantium bergamia*)
Recommended dilution: ½% to 1%
Bergamot orange essential oil should not be confused with the common herbaceous plant Monarda, which is also known as bergamot. The essential oil is produced from a pear-shaped orange that is grown primarily for its peel and the oil therein. It has a citrus-floral scent that is pleasant, although the essential oil is a powerful antiseptic. It is effective on dry skin; there is an uplifting quality about it. Use with care, however, as exposure to sun after the application of bergamot orange essential oil can cause skin pigmentation.

BLACK PEPPER
(*Piper nigrum*)
Recommended dilution: ½% to 1%
This common kitchen spice makes a subtle yet powerful oil. It is warming in small amounts and is highly recommended for treating colds, flu, chills and painful coughs. Combines well with frankincense and marjoram essential oils.

CAMOMILE, GERMAN

(*Matricaria chamomilla*)

Recommended dilution: 1% to 3%

German camomile is the common herb-tea ingredient that was used to settle Peter Rabbit's upset tummy. When it is massaged onto the belly, German camomile essential oil in a dilution has the same soothing effect—on the liver as well as the rest of the digestive system. It also helps relieve sore muscles and bruises and is good for sensitive skin. You can add this camomile to shampoos and rinses for fair hair.

CAMOMILE, ROMAN

(*Anthemis nobile*)

Recommended dilution: ½% to 1%

Roman camomile is very different from German camomile. It smells sweet, almost like apples. It is anti-inflammatory and useful for treating skin problems related to sensitivity, irritations, redness, and so on.

CAMPHOR

(*Cinnamomum camphora*)

Recommended dilution: 1%

The mild scent of camphor essential oil is misleading, as it is a powerful antiseptic that can be toxic if overused. When first applied to the skin, it may feel slightly cool, but the effect soon changes to a warming sensation. Good for treating acne and oily skin, bruises, rheumatic inflammations and fevers.

CYPRESS

(*Cupressus sempervirens*)

Recommended dilution: 1%

Mildly toning, styptic and diuretic, cypress is good for treating oily skin and acne, varicose veins and water retention. This essential oil is also mildly stimulating for the circulation.

EUCALYPTUS

(*Eucalyptus* spp)

Recommended dilution: 1% to 5%

Even if you're not familiar with essential oils in general, chances are you've come into contact with eucalyptus essential oil. It has been widely used in chest and muscle rubs and is often added to the water in vaporizers and humidifiers to purify the air. Having antiseptic and antibacterial properties, eucalyptus essential oil is also effective in destroying airborne staphylococci. It is mild and, in dilution, is effective for treating colds, headaches, sinus congestion, muscular aches and pains, joint aches and fever.

FRANKINCENSE

(*Boswellia carteri*)

Recommended dilution: 1% to 3%

The oil obtained by distilling the gum of trees of the genus *Boswellia* is a common component of church incense. It is antiseptic and warming, making it useful in the treatment of chills, colds, respiratory congestion and indigestion. For skin care, it is toning and restorative.

GERANIUM

(*Pelargonium* spp)

Recommended dilution: 1% to 3%

Geranium is a neutral oil, much like lavender, which makes it useful for extreme skin conditions, such as oily or dry skin and eczema. It helps in the regeneration of skin that has been burned, cut or bruised and cools inflammations. Refreshing for general skin care.

GRAPEFRUIT

(*Citrus paradisi*)

See Lemon.

JASMINE

(*Jasminum officinale*)

Recommended dilution: ½% to 1%

Real jasmine essential oil by steam distillation is no longer available commercially. The oil is usually obtained by maceration or extraction by solvents. It has a lovely scent and many benefits. Jasmine is warming and uplifting and is toning for hot, dry skin.

JUNIPER
(*Juniperus communis*)

Recommended dilution: 1% to 3%

The same juniper berry that flavours gin makes an interesting oil which is warming, astringent, antiseptic and diuretic. For acne or oily skin, it is good in a facial oil or compress. As a bath additive or massage oil, it helps alleviate fluid retention and is also used for treating rheumatism and aching joints.

LAVENDER
(*Lavandula officinalis*)

Recommended dilution: 1% to 5%

If you must choose just one essential oil, make it lavender. Lavender essential oil is a fairly neutral oil, which means that its effects on the skin are neither hot nor cold. This quality makes it the only essential oil which can be used neat, or uncut, on the skin and which is perfectly safe for children. Don't let that lull you into thinking that lavender essential oil is not potent, however. Antiseptic and balancing, it can be used to treat extremes such as very dry or oily skin, and it helps lower high blood pressure as well as stimulate a sluggish system. Keep a dilution handy to use on insect stings, burns and scalds, inflammations of any kind, minor cuts and scrapes, blemishes, and so on. Beware the synthetic lavender on the market, which is characterized by a sweet, cloying fragrance. Genuine lavender has a fresh, clean scent.

LEMON
(*Citrus limon*)

Also: Grapefruit, Lime, Mandarin, Orange, Tangerine

Recommended dilution: 1% to 5%

Lemon and the other citrus essential oils are fairly similar, so I've addressed them together. They are all diuretic, astringent and antiseptic and are useful for toning oily skin and for treating water retention. A few drops mixed into a shampoo or conditioner will help an oily scalp and bring out the sheen in fair hair. These oils are relatively inexpensive but do not store well. Buy in small quantities as needed, or store in a dark, cool place. If they turn cloudy, discard. Adding a little vegetable oil such as sunflower, peanut, rice bran or grape-seed (at about 10 percent of the volume of the essential oil) will help stabilize them.

LIME
(*Citrus aurantifolia*)

See Lemon.

MANDARIN
(*Citrus nobilis*)

See Lemon.

MARJORAM
(*Origanum majorana*)

Recommended dilution:
1% to 3%

Marjoram seems to combine a floral, herbal and camphoraceous scent. It is antiseptic, soothing and warming, making it a good rub for rheumatic pains, muscular aches, bruises, colds and sinus congestion. It is often blended with orange essential oil, but for a warming winter oil, I like it with frankincense or black pepper essential oil.

Juniper
Juniperus communis

MELISSA

(*Melissa officinalis*)

Recommended dilution: 1% to 5%

As a herb, its more common name is lemon balm, but whatever you call it, melissa makes a delightful addition to any garden. Its essential oil, however, is very volatile and delicate, and a fair amount of herb is required to produce the oil. As a result, most melissa essential oil on the market is mingled with lemongrass or citronella essential oil, both of which are significantly cheaper. Because of its antispasmodic qualities, pure melissa essential oil can be used to treat tension and nervousness. It is also mildly warming.

MYRRH

(*Commiphora myrrha*)

Recommended dilution: 1% to 2%

The gum from myrrh makes a dark, resinous oil that is excellent for toning mature skin and for treating scars, infections, acne, dermatitis and a variety of mouth problems, such as cankers and gum inflammation. (See also Myrrh Tincture in The Pharmacy.)

NEROLI

(*Citrus aurantium*)

Recommended dilution: ½%

Like most of the citrus essential oils, pure neroli is toning for oily skin and is beneficial for mature skin too. It is most useful, however, as a soothing and calming agent for the nervous system. Pure neroli essential oil is very expensive.

ORANGE

(*Citrus sinensis*)

See Lemon.

PATCHOULI

(*Pogostemon cablin*)

Recommended dilution: 1% to 3%

The warm, earthy scent of patchouli became a popular perfume fragrance in North America during the 1960s and 1970s. It is a mild antiseptic and is useful for dry, cracked skin, acne and eczema. A few drops mixed into a shampoo or conditioner will condition the scalp and highlight dark hair.

PEPPERMINT

(*Mentha piperita*)

Recommended dilution: ½% to 3%

Peppermint is a familiar taste to most people; it is used in toothpastes, mouthwashes, breath mints, flavourings, tea, and so on. The skin's first reaction to peppermint is a cooling sensation. Use it to stimulate a sluggish circulation or to treat bruises, swelling, headaches, nausea, sore feet and tired legs. But remember to go easy—too much peppermint can irritate.

PETITGRAIN

(*Citrus aurantium*)

Recommended dilution: 1% to 3%

If you find the cost of pure neroli essential oil prohibitive, try petitgrain essential oil as a substitute. It is distilled from the leaves of the same tree that produces neroli (made from orange blossoms) Although not as potent as neroli, petitgrain has similar qualities and a pleasant fragrance and is significantly cheaper. Mildly diuretic and stimulating.

ROSE

(*Rosa* spp)

Recommended dilution: ½% to 1%

According to *A Modern Herbal* by Mrs. M. Grieve, it takes over 8,800 pounds (4,000 kg) of fresh roses to make just a couple of pounds (1 kg) of essential oil. As a result, pure rose essential oil is one of the most costly oils—and one of the most potent. It has an incredible fragrance and is an important healing substance. It helps the skin retain its elasticity and is used to treat sensitive and mature skin as well as redness, dryness and broken capillaries.

ROSEMARY

(*Rosmarinus officinalis*)

Recommended dilution: 1% to 3%

Warming and stimulating, rosemary essential oil is used in massage oils for rheumatic pain, muscular aches and sluggish circulation. It is toning and emollient and is therefore effective in treating dandruff and scalp conditions and for toning normal and oily skin.

SANDALWOOD

(*Santalum album*)

Recommended dilution: 1% to 5%

This heavy, mild oil is excellent for very dry skin conditions and inflammations. For use on dry, red, itchy, cracked or chapped skin, blend it with lighter essential oils, such as lavender, geranium or petitgrain. Sandalwood is also an effective antiseptic.

SPRUCE

(*Picea* spp)

Recommended dilution: 1% to 5%

The old saying "spruced up" is a fair description of the effects of this oil. Spruce essential oil can be easily confused with balsam fir essential oil, but its action is more lively, warming and uplifting. It is especially good for the legs and feet.

TANGERINE

(*Citrus reticulata*)

See Lemon.

YLANG-YLANG

(*Cananga odorata*)

Recommended dilution: ½% to 1%

Ylang-ylang is a tropical flower with a heavy fragrance. It has a soothing, relaxing effect on the skin and nervous system. I find that on its own, though, its scent is too sweet. It is best used in a blend with an essential oil such as geranium, sandalwood or one of the citrus oils. Use sparingly.

METHODS & EQUIPMENT

Science means simply the aggregate of all the recipes that are always successful. The rest is literature.
—Paul Valéry

Whether the result is for consumption or for external application, every recipe demands a range of skills from the "cook." The cook might also need a bit of magic, some "literature" and a little *je ne sais quoi*. Over the years, I have attempted many different methods for processing natural ingredients and creating concoctions that can be used for skin and hair care. Some have worked, while some have been dismal failures, regardless of my frame of mind when I made them or how many times I tried. To create even the humble omelette, you must follow a prescribed method. But what produces a light, fluffy dish one day might result in

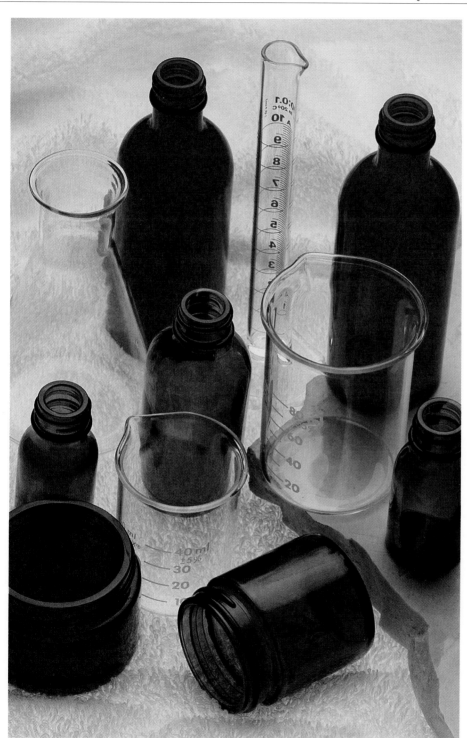

Equipment needs for making skin-care items are simple and inexpensive.

a decidedly unappetizing meal the next. In this chapter, I will share the methods that have worked most effectively for me, with or without the help of serendipity.

There are a few very basic methods for processing natural skin-care ingredients, and once you know them, you can duplicate the processes whenever you choose. It's much like learning to make a good omelette. At a certain point, there's no further need for instruction, only inspiration and a little *je ne sais quoi*.

METHODS

Although you can purchase many of the ingredients called for in these recipes in a pharmacy or a natural-food store, it is easy to make some of them yourself, especially if you have the time and the plant materials on hand. Before trying any of these methods, please refer to the chapter "Ingredients" to determine the characteristics of the plants you want to use. Many of the methods discussed here involve a solvent, such as alcohol, water or oil, that is used to extract the beneficial properties of the herbs. Although that process may sound a little daunting, anybody who has brewed a pot of tea has made an aqueous—or liquid—extract. In that case, the properties of the herb—tea—have been infused into a solvent—boiling water—to create a comforting drink. It's that simple.

TINCTURES

A tincture is produced when we subject plant material to a solvent—usually alcohol or vinegar—in order to extract the plant's central components and so render them usable for external applications. The result is a potent liquid product that is convenient and easy to use. Tinctures are an ingredient in many skin-care recipes—among them, facial toners, creams and lotions.

Although the method involved in making a tincture is similar to that for making, say, a herbal tea, the use of alcohol as the solvent allows some plant compounds to be dissolved and held in the alcohol that might not be released by merely steeping herbs in boiling water (essential oils, for instance).

If you do not want to use alcohol as the solvent, vinegar can be substituted. However, a vinegar-based tincture lasts only a year, while an alcohol-based tincture will last for several. My preference is for grain alcohol, although vodka and brandy are common choices as well. Whatever alcoholic solvent you choose, it should be at least 40 percent alcohol by volume; the vinegar should be at least 5 percent by volume, although 7 percent pickling vinegar is better. Do not use rubbing alcohol. Its scent is overpowering, and it can have a very drying effect on some skin types.

To make a tincture, chop one or two handfuls of clean, dry plant material into bits about ¼ to 1 inch in length. Although a blender or a food processor can do this chopping, using a knife will decrease the amount of essential oil lost from the plant through overhandling. With a delicate herb such as lemon balm, chop coarsely and gently. If the part of the plant called for is the berry, root or bark, crush lightly.

Place the plant material in a clean glass jar with a tight-fitting lid, and add enough alcohol or vinegar to submerge the material completely. Then cover the jar, and leave in a dark place for six to eight weeks. Shake the jar every few days, and check the contents. Top up with more alcohol or vinegar if it is being absorbed by the plant material.

At the end of this period, filter the contents of the jar through a fine-mesh screen or several layers of cheesecloth. You can also use unbleached coffee filters. Squeeze the remaining liquid from the herbs before you discard them. Store the tincture in a clean glass jar, preferably dark glass with a dropper.

INFUSIONS

Making an infusion is, simply, making a tea. Pouring boiling water over chopped or crushed plant material and allowing it to steep will yield the useful properties of most plants to the water.

To make an infusion mild enough to be used directly on the skin, use 1 Tbsp. (15 mL) dried herb *or* ¼ cup (50 mL) fresh herb for every 1 cup (250 mL) boiling water. You can wait until the infusion is either tepid or cool before straining the herb out and using the liquid. To make a very strong infusion, or "brew," use just enough boiling water to cover the herb.

The beneficial properties of certain roots, dried berries, bark, thick-leaved plants and seeds will be released if you gently simmer them in water for 5 to 10 minutes. To make these infusions, use 1 tsp. (5 mL) plant material to every 1 cup (250 mL) water.

Plant materials, such as comfrey or marshmallow root, that contain mucilage (see "Plant Directory" in the chapter "Ingredients") or other sugars should be infused with tepid or cold water, because boiling water will cause their sugars to break down, rendering them less effec-tive. Add water to the herb, using the same proportions as you would to make a regular hot infusion. Cover, and let the mixture stand for a few hours. If you are using cold water, mash the plant a little in the water to help the process along. Strain well.

To store infusions, place in a covered container and refrigerate. Use within a few days. They will keep for a week or so if you add ¼ tsp. (1 mL) citric acid or the juice of a quarter of a lemon, strained, to every 1 cup (250 mL) infusion.

WASH

A wash is a mild infusion that is "washed" over the skin. Gently pour or mist the infusion onto the part of the skin you wish to treat.

MACERATION

To macerate plant material is to reduce it to a pulp using water. Coarsely chop plant material, preferably fresh, and place in a sturdy bowl or large mortar. Add small amounts of cold, tepid or hot water, depending on the effect you want, and mash until the material is a nondescript mass. (Cold water should be used for macerations made to treat swelling; tepid water for rashes, scrapes, dryness, eczema and hives; and hot water for chills, congestion and pulled muscles.) The material should be moist but not watery. Macerated plant material can be used for poultices.

POULTICE

My grandmother used mustard plasters to ease the discomfort experienced by my grandfather, who had been gassed during World War I. She mixed mustard and flour with enough water to make a paste, sandwiched the mixture between two pieces of flannel that had been soaked in hot water and laid the whole thing on his chest. The heat helped the volatile oil of the mustard to penetrate and so ease the congestion in his lungs. This is one method of using a poultice.

The same principles apply when you are making a poultice with macerated herbs or an infusion. The temperature you use depends on the effect you want (see "Maceration," previous page). Use cheesecloth, gauze, cotton or cotton flannel to hold the herbs or the infusion. Put a thin layer of the macerated herbs on a cloth, and cover with a second layer of cloth, or completely soak two layers of cloth in an infusion and place on the afflicted area. Leave for 5 to 10 minutes, then change the herbs or resoak in the infusion. Do this for 20 to 30 minutes.

INFUSED OIL

When reading these recipes or when buying ingredients, be careful not to confuse infused oils with essential oils. An essential oil is the volatile aromatic oil that is derived from a plant by steam distillation (see the chapter "Ingredients" for a more complete discussion). Although many herbs—calendula, for instance—do not produce an essential oil, their benefits can nevertheless be infused into a vegetable oil in a process that is similar to making a water infusion. These infused oils can then be used in a variety of skin-care items, such as massage oils, creams and ointments.

Some instructions for infusing oils recommend letting the herbs sit in oil for a week or two before straining. Many herbs contain a lot of moisture that remains in the oil when you use this technique. That moisture can cause the oil to turn rancid within a short period of time.

I have developed the following method to avoid that problem.

Coarsely chop several handfuls of fresh herbs, and place in a heavy stainless steel pot. Cover with an inexpensive olive oil. Gently heat the oil until the herbs are wilted, remove from heat, and let cool, uncovered. (Some people recommend heating the oil until the herbs become crispy. This gives a "deep-fried" quality to the oil that I do not like; I suspect that it also destroys some of the plant's constituent properties.) Let the wilted plant sit in the oil for a few hours or overnight. Strain well, removing all bits of plant material. Most of the moisture from the plant will have separated from the oil, just as oil and vinegar in a salad dressing will separate. Simply "decant," or pour off, the oil into another pan. Gently heat the oil again. As the remaining moisture evaporates, each droplet will rise to the surface of the oil and burst into a tiny spray. When the droplets have stopped bursting, the oil is free of water content. This process can take up to an hour or two. Let the oil cool completely. Decant into a bottle, and label with plant used and date made. (To decant, slowly pour the oil into another container, taking care not to disturb any sediment remaining on the bottom. When the sediment starts to unsettle, stop pouring and discard what is left in the pot.)

It is also possible to use dried plant material when creating an infused oil, although some of the benefits won't be quite as apparent as they are with fresh herbs. Coarsely chop clean, dry plant material, and cover with olive oil. Gently heat for a few minutes, then let cool completely. Strain so that all bits of herbs are removed. Decant into a bottle, and label as above.

BAIN-MARIE, OR WATER-BATH

When the recipe calls for the ingredients to be heated, as in the preparation of ointments and creams, you will need a bain-marie, or water-bath. Using a bain-marie prevents the overheating of delicate natural ingredients and keeps water-based ingredients from evaporating.

To create a bain-marie, use either a stainless steel double boiler or a smaller pot that fits into a larger one containing hot water. The smaller pot should touch the water. Using this method, you can heat and melt oils, waxes and fats without "frying" them. While ingredients such as beeswax and lanolin require a stove (medium heat so that the water is very hot but not boiling), other liquids, such as liquid honey, tinctures and infusions, need only be placed in a small bowl that is in turn fitted into a larger bowl containing hot water.

EQUIPMENT

You don't need to set up a home laboratory to make your own skin-care products. You probably already have much of the equipment you will need in your kitchen. The most important consideration should be that your equipment and surroundings are clean. Anything that comes into contact with what you're creating should be washed in hot, soapy water and rinsed. The counter or table upon which you work should be scrupulously clean.

The equipment you will need is markedly unromantic. Forget wooden spoons and quaint cracked crocks; their porous texture allows them to absorb and retain

residue from the ingredients. Stainless steel and glass are the ideal materials for creating homemade skin-care items, because they can be easily and thoroughly cleaned. Use soap and hot water for cleaning, followed by a wipe with a cloth doused in alcohol—rubbing alcohol is fine—then a good rinse in hot water. If you are making creams or ointments, sterilize your glass jars and containers by placing them in a cold oven and heating to 200 degrees F (93°C) for 30 minutes. If you are using plastic, completely immerse the containers and lids in water that has come to a rolling boil, and leave for five minutes. Then allow the pieces to air-dry.

The following list contains specific equipment suggestions, but feel free to substitute anything else that you have in your cupboard, keeping in mind the need for a surface that is impenetrable.

GRADUATED CYLINDERS

Available in many sizes, the smaller graduated cylinders are well suited for making home cosmetics. The 10 mL size, with 1 mL increments marked on the side, is ideal for essential oils, while the 50 mL to 100 mL size should be used when measuring oils and other liquids. If they are not available at your pharmacy or local hobby shop, they can probably be ordered.

BEAKERS

More squat than cylinders, beakers are less likely to topple over. Although measurements for tiny amounts are not marked on them, beakers are fine for measuring larger quantities of liquid or dry ingredients. I recommend a 50 mL or 100 mL to 150 mL beaker for making home cosmetics.

GLASS MEASURING CUP

A good-quality measuring cup—the kind you would use in cooking. Be sure it is glass and measures in cup and/or 25 mL increments.

GLASS MEDICINE DROPPERS

For measuring essential oils. Clean thoroughly after use so as not to contaminate other oils.

GOGGLES

If you are working with essential oils, wearing protective eye gear will guard against accidental splashes.

APRON OR OLD CLOTHES

Especially when working with oils.

RAGS

For cleanup.

TISSUE PAPER OR NEWSPAPER

I usually put down several layers of newspaper first, followed by a few sheets of tissue paper to protect the surface I'm working on, removing the layers of tissue if they become too wet or messy.

BOTTLES AND JARS

It is always handy to have a selection of containers from which to choose. Coloured glass is best for storing skin-care products, because it diffuses light. Amber glass can often be purchased in pharmacies or in stores that sell bulk items. Although green and blue glass bottles are very pretty and make lovely containers for gift-giving, they're harder to come by and more expensive.

Otherwise, feel free to use recycled containers, as long as they originally held either an edible or a cosmetic substance. Soak off any labels, then clean thoroughly by washing in hot, soapy water and rinsing well several times or by sterilizing according to the methods described on the previous page. Don't forget to clean caps and lids too. While it is acceptable to put glass items in the dishwasher, I would be somewhat more cautious about plastic containers. A recycled plastic container can be deodorized by swishing it with a half-and-half mixture of vinegar and water and 1 Tbsp. (15 mL) baking soda, letting it soak for a while, then rinsing well. (If it still has a significant odour after that, take it to the recycling depot.) I store bulk quantities in large glass or food-grade plastic containers, refilling small ones for everyday use. Here are a few suggestions for containers that may be recycled for specific skin-care products:

Shampoo, Conditioner or Bubble-Bath Bottles: For bath items.

Cream or Petroleum-Jelly Jars: For creams and ointments, especially if they're not too big and haven't previously held something strongly scented.

Tiny Jam Jars: For smaller quantities of creams and ointments.

Vinegar Bottles: For body and facial vinegars.

Glass Vegetable-Oil Bottles: For massage and bath oils.

A good source for such items as amber glass bottles, glass eyedroppers, dropper bottles and plastic squeeze bottles is your local pharmacy. Pharmacies usually stock these items to use when filling prescriptions. If they are not on hand, they can be ordered, although you may have to buy a minimum of six or a dozen. (You might want to explain how you intend to use them. When I used to buy quantities of small vials for essential oils, I was constantly kidded about being a drug dealer.)

Some natural-food stores stock empty bottles, especially if they sell bulk items, as do mail-order companies that deal in essential oils or food items. If you're looking for more attractive jars for gift-giving, check out flea markets and secondhand stores for sound, uncracked jars or look in the kitchen or bath section of department or gift stores for inexpensive jars that can be made attractive with a piece of ribbon and a label. Don't forget to give yourself one too.

THE BATH

I have had a good many more uplifting thoughts, creative and expansive visions, while soaking in comfortable baths or drying myself after bracing showers …than I have ever had in any cathedral.
—Edmund Wilson, *A Piece of My Mind*

It's true that the pretensions and extravagances of life can sometimes leave an individual feeling insignificant, but I suspect that Edmund Wilson's visions might not have been quite so expansive without the glory of a cathedral to reflect upon, in the bath or anywhere else. Yet it's hard to deny that one of the most beneficial and pleasant routines we can incorporate into our lives is the bath, that private place where we can truly get a sense of ourselves. I have discovered that it is one of the few places where I can actually listen to myself breathe. Still, most of us continue to jump into a shower, wash our hair and bodies and

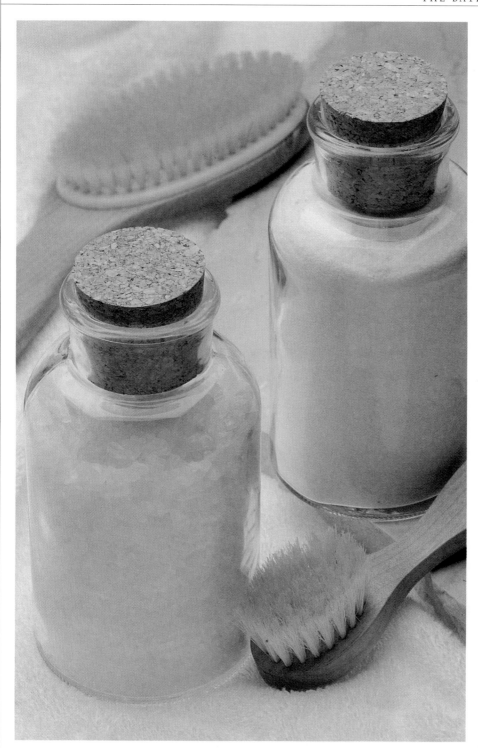

*Coarse and
refined sea salts
make excellent
bath additives.*

hop out. Cleaning ourselves has become a perfunctory affair, rather than a time for contemplation. And modern bathtubs seem to be nothing more than larger-than-usual shower stalls. What a shame! A sweetly scented bath can be not only soothing to the skin but comforting to the soul as well.

When I started my own business, I was driven, like so many of the self-employed, to burn the candle at both ends. I paid for this inattention to my mental and physical needs by spending almost an entire winter sick in bed, as my weakened and stressed-out immune system offered a welcoming environment to each opportunistic virus that was making the rounds. I eventually came to understand that taking time out for recreation which refreshed and relaxed me did not have to reduce my productivity.

The responsibilities of modern life—family, work, school, deadlines, bills, household chores and a dozen other obligations that demand our energies—seem to conspire against the self-reflective bath. The truth is that pampering ourselves doesn't have to take long, and we inevitably emerge better able to deal with the pressures which sent us there in the first place. These days, my favourite treat of all is to draw myself a hot bath and settle in to listen to myself breathe, while I let the answering machine take my messages. A 20-minute bath can be an essential time-out for which we need feel no guilt; everything will still be waiting for us when we step out.

BATH BASICS

Bathwater should be at a slightly higher temperature than your body but never so hot that you look like a cooked lobster when you emerge. If you are suffering from a fever or from some sort of inflamed-skin condition, a cool bath is in order. The recommended length for any bath, hot or cool, however, is 20 minutes. After that, your fingers and toes begin to shrivel up like raisins.

Before you bathe or shower, a quick brush over your skin with a dry loofah or a natural-bristle brush will help keep the skin fresh, loosen the dead cells and stimulate circulation. Brush your skin using small, light strokes, going over any one spot only two or three times and avoiding troubled or broken areas. Always stroke toward the heart, going with the flow of the surface circulation. Your skin should be pink after a dry-brush. If it's screaming red, you've overdone it.

If you are especially oily, sweaty or dirty, have a quick shower before settling into a bath.

OATMEAL BATH

Oatmeal is one of the best ingredients for treating dry, sensitive skin. When I was a child and suffered from hives, my mother gave me tepid oatmeal baths that helped soothe the itching. Oatmeal is also very effective for eczema, psoriasis, chicken pox and other skin eruptions.

For one bath, use ½ to 1 cup (125-250 mL) oatmeal that has been pounded in a mortar or whizzed in a blender until it is a fine powder. If you're short on time, use ½ cup (125 mL) oatmeal flour, which is already in powdered form. Sprinkle the powder into the bathwater, and soak for 20 minutes, rubbing any floating powder onto the skin. Pat yourself dry. If you are treating a skin ailment, keep the bath-water tepid or cool.

You can also substitute ½ cup (125 mL) rolled oats tied in a square of cheesecloth or muslin. While this method is not as effective as putting the oatmeal directly into the water, it provides similar benefits.

HONEY AND OATMEAL BATH ✓

The combination of soothing oatmeal and the moisturizing benefits of honey is an effective treatment for dry, itchy skin or for sensitive or mature skin.

For one bath, use ¼ to ½ cup (50-125 mL) ground rolled oats, employing the same method as that used in Oatmeal Bath. Dissolve 1 Tbsp. to ¼ cup (15-50 mL) honey in warm water, then add to the bath.

BARLEY AND OATMEAL BATH

This bath preparation is very emollient and soothing. You can substitute short-grain rice for the barley.

In 8 cups (2 L) water, gently simmer ¼ cup (50 mL) pearl barley and ¼ cup (50 mL) rolled oats for 20 minutes. Strain, and add the cooking water to the bath.

HERBAL OATMEAL BATH

This preparation offers the emollience of oatmeal as well as the refreshing effects of herbs.

Mix ¼ cup (50 mL) rolled oats with a small handful of mixed herbs, such as lavender, rose petals, spearmint, camomile, scented geranium or thyme. (See "Herbal Baths," page 48, for further suggestions.) Tie mixture in a square of cheesecloth, and toss into the bath.

SALT BATHS

Salt is an excellent bath additive for sore, aching muscles as well as a number of skin complaints, such as psoriasis, eczema and minor rashes. Use ¼ to 1 cup (50-250 mL) of any of the following:

common kitchen salt, sea salt, unrefined sea salt, Epsom salts or pickling salt. If you're really in a bad way, you can use up to 2 cups (500 mL) of salt in a bath.

After a bath this potent, however, you will probably feel slightly enervated, so wrap up warmly, and lie down and rest.

BATH SALTS ✓
FOR HARD WATER

A heaping tablespoon of this mixture sprinkled into the bath softens the water, but using all of it will put you to sleep!

Combine ½ cup (125 mL) Epsom salts, ¼ cup (50 mL) baking soda and ¼ tsp. (1 mL) borax. Mix well, and store in a covered container.

SCENTED BATH SALTS ✓

Scented bath salts are easy to make, and dressed up in a preserving jar or a similar container, they are appealing gifts. For a quantity of bath salts that will give you pleasure through many baths, sprinkle 2 cups (500 mL) coarse sea salt or pickling salt with 20 to 40 drops of a pure essential oil. Blend thoroughly. You can combine more than one essential oil (see "Bath Oils"), but do not exceed 40 drops in total. For more exotic-looking bath salts, blend in a few drops of vegetable food colouring. Store mixture in a tightly covered glass container away from direct

Wild Rose
Rosa spp

light. For one bath, use ¼ cup (50 mL). If you choose to use one essential oil rather than a blend of oils, I recommend the following: bergamot orange, camomile, eucalyptus, pure jasmine, juniper, lavender, lemon, lime, mandarin, orange, peppermint, petitgrain, pure rose, rose geranium, rosemary, sandalwood or tangerine.

MILK BATHS

With these simple recipes, you can take advantage of an ingredient you're sure to have on hand.

MILK BATH

Milk is a gentle and effective skin cleanser. Add 1 to 2 cups (250-500 mL) milk to the bath. For dry skin, use a high-butterfat milk or an equal combination of milk and cream. For oily skin, use skim milk or buttermilk. You can also use ⅓ cup (75 mL) milk powder (the instant kind works best). And if you want a truly refreshing experience, throw in ¼ cup (50 mL) Epsom salts or baking soda with the milk.

HERBAL MILK BATH

Soaking in a sweetly scented herbal milk bath is a soothing way to cleanse and rejuvenate the skin.

In 1 to 2 cups (250-500 mL) milk, steep a handful or two of any of the following herbs in the refrigerator overnight (or gently heat together till just warm, then cool): borage leaves, calendula flowers, elder flowers, lavender flowers, lemon verbena, lemon thyme, fragrant roses, scented-geranium leaves, spearmint or sweet violets. After steeping, mash the herbs thoroughly, strain, then add milk to the bath.

MILK AND ALMOND BATH

In a blender, mix together ½ cup (125 mL) milk and 1 Tbsp. to ¼ cup (15-50 mL) ground almonds, which are an effective skin softener. Let sit for an hour or overnight in the refrigerator. Strain, and add milk to the bath.

SILK BATH

This bath has a softening and rejuvenating effect on the skin.

Blend ⅓ cup (75 mL) powdered milk, 1 tsp. (5 mL) orrisroot powder and ¼ cup (50 mL) salt, removing any lumps. Sprinkle into running water.

HERBAL BATHS

When I was in the business of creating and selling my own herbal concoctions, one of the most popular items was a bath mix of rose, lavender, comfrey root, spearmint, thyme, violet leaves and hibiscus blended with essential oils of pure rose, lavender and pure jasmine. I stored it for a few weeks, making a potpourri of sorts, then sold it in a cotton drawstring bag. A customer who was going through a rocky period said that on one particularly bad day, she had retreated to the bath with this mixture. "It changed my life," she insisted.

That claim might be a little extravagant, but the soothing effect of this herbal combination almost certainly helped my

Borage
Borago
officinalis

client out from under an overwhelming moment. And I'm sure it was better for her than a pharmaceutical sedative or a quick belt of Scotch.

Please Note: Never use commercial potpourris for herbal baths. Many contain synthetic fragrances that are not intended for use on the skin. Even homemade potpourris may contain spices and certain oils that will irritate the skin.

Basic Directions: Creating a herbal bath can be as simple as wandering into the garden, gathering up a few sprigs of herbs, tying them in a square of cheesecloth and tossing it into the bathwater. If you don't have a garden, fresh herbs from the grocer or good-quality dried herbs are an acceptable substitute. When fresh herbs are available, use one to two large handfuls per bath. If you are using dried herbs, a cupped handful will do.

You can steep the herbs as you would for tea and strain before adding the liquid to the bath. As an alternative, I like to tie the herbs loosely in a square of cheesecloth or a reusable muslin drawstring bag and hang it under the running water as I am drawing my bath. Once in the bath, I squeeze the bag over me and rub it lightly on my skin. Follow these basic directions to prepare each of the recipes below.

BATH HERBS FOR DRY SKIN

These herbs are emollient and/or soothing and should be used when treating sunburned skin, dry or cracked skin, and so on. Following Basic Directions outlined above, use one of *or* a combination of: self-heal, speedwell, calendula flowers, comfrey leaf or root, heartsease (Johnny-jump-up), mallow leaves, marshmallow root, plantain leaves and seeds, rosebuds and rose petals, Roman camomile flowers or scented-geranium leaves.

SOOTHING BATH HERBS

Used according to Basic Directions, any of these herbs, alone or in combination, are wonderful for calming the nerves and aiding in relaxation (they are also suitable for sensitive skin): camomile flowers, lavender flowers, lemon verbena leaves, lemon balm, linden flowers, rose petals, spearmint leaves or valerian root.

BATH HERBS FOR TONING

Use one of *or* a combination of these herbs according to Basic Directions to tone and strengthen the skin and to treat bruises and sore, tired legs and feet: basil, ground ivy, horsetail, hyssop, juniper berries, nettle, rosemary, southernwood or yarrow.

HERBAL BATH FOR SORE MUSCLES

If you're aching all over, these herbs are a perfect antidote. They are also an effective treatment for bruises and are soothing when you feel a chill coming on. Use one of *or* a combination of the following according to Basic Directions: bay leaves, birch leaves, eucalyptus leaves, the pulverized seed of horse chestnut, marjoram, sage, St.-John's-wort, thyme or wild marjoram.

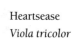

Heartsease
Viola tricolor

CORDIAL BATH HERBS

These are "cordial" herbs, renowned for their cooling and soothing properties, especially with irritated skin. They are also mildly deodorant.

Use one of *or* a combination of the following according to Basic Directions: angelica root, borage leaves, chickweed, cleavers, lavender, lovage root, orrisroot, sweet clover or sweet violet.

'SLIMMING' BATH HERBS

A combination of these herbs will help draw out impurities from normal and oily skin as well as tone it. They are especially effective for those who are dieting or fasting; some people even recommend them as a treatment for hangovers. Use one of *or* a combination of the following according to Basic Directions: burdock or yellow dock root, citrus peels, dandelion root, echinacea root, fennel seeds, juniper berries, kelp or bladder wrack, nettle, parsley or red clover.

This bath is made even more effective with the addition of 1 cup (250 mL) salt (see "Salt Baths").

Hyssop
*Hyssopus
officinalis*

BATH OILS

The heat of the bath helps to open the pores, thereby allowing bath oils to penetrate and be assimilated by the skin. These oils are easy to make and very effective; one drawback is the slight ring they leave around the tub after you have drained the water. Simply clean the tub right away, and that won't be a problem.

These oils can be mixed in equal proportions with a dispersing "oil"—grain alcohol, vodka or brandy—but if you use this method, be sure to shake the mixture well before adding it to the bath. Some British reference books recommend using sulphonated castor oil, which is also known as Turkey-red oil, because it will disperse in water. Unfortunately, I have been unable to discover a North American source.

EASIEST BATH OIL ✓
IN THE WORLD

This is one of the simplest and most inexpensive treats you can give yourself, and it is effective as well. Just add 1 to 2 tsp. (5-10 mL) olive, sweet almond, sunflower, peanut or apricot kernel oil to the bathwater, and hop in.

SUPEREMOLLIENT BATH OIL

A bath in this oil will leave your skin supple as well as moist, and it is especially effective with dry skin. The addition of alcohol helps the oil to disperse.

1 cup (250 mL) sweet almond, olive, apricot kernel or another rich oil
2 Tbsp. (30 mL) castor, wheat germ or avocado oil
1 tsp. (5 mL) anhydrous lanolin
½ cup (125 mL) vodka or grain alcohol (optional)
20 drops sandalwood or geranium essential oil *or* 5 drops pure rose essential oil (optional)

Gently heat the first three ingredients in a heavy saucepan or a double boiler until the lanolin melts. If adding alcohol, whisk it into the oil at this point. When mixture is cool, blend in essential oil. Bottle and label. Shake well before adding to bathwater. Use only 1 tsp. (5 mL) per bath.

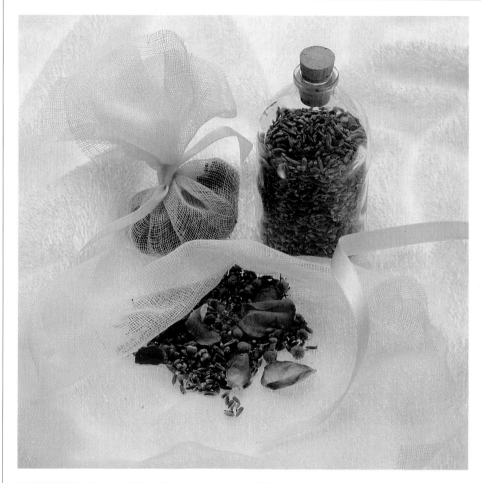

Herbal bath sachets of soothing bath herbs feature lavender, rose petals and camomile.

LUXURIOUS BATH OIL

Intended for normal to very dry skin, this bath oil coats the skin and is assimilated well.

¼ cup (50 mL) comfrey or plantain infused oil or plain olive oil

¼ cup (50 mL) sesame oil (not the toasted kind)

½ cup (125 mL) sweet almond or apricot kernel oil

¼ cup (50 mL) avocado or castor oil

20 drops pure jasmine, bergamot orange or ylang-ylang essential oil (optional)

Swirl together until blended. Bottle and label. Use 1 to 2 tsp. (5-10 mL) per bath.

HERBAL BATH OILS

A simple bath oil is an infused herbal oil. (To learn how to infuse oil, see chapter "Methods & Equipment.") Depending on the effect you want, use any of the following herbal bath oils singly or in combination: borage, calendula, camomile, comfrey, marshmallow, mallow, plantain, rosemary, scented geranium, southernwood or yarrow. Use 1 to 2 tsp. (5-10 mL) per bath.

SCENTED BATH OILS

A little bottle containing a scented bath oil that you have created yourself makes

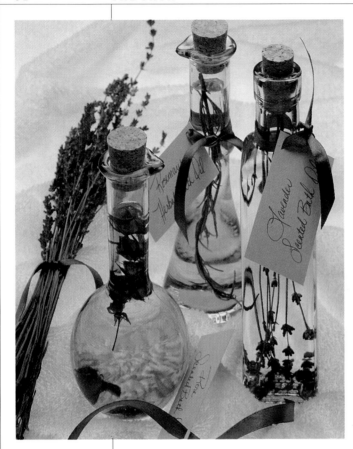

Rosemary herbal, lavender- and rose-scented bath oils.

SCENTED BATH OIL FOR SENSITIVE SKIN

To 1 cup (250 mL) rice bran or grape-seed oil, add 10 drops pure rose essential oil *or* 60 drops camomile or lavender essential oil. Swirl together until well blended. Use 1 to 2 tsp. (5-10 mL) per bath.

SCENTED BATH OIL FOR MATURE SKIN

To 1 cup (250 mL) apricot kernel or sunflower oil, add 40 drops lavender essential oil, 20 drops petitgrain or bergamot orange essential oil and 10 drops ylang-ylang essential oil (optional). Swirl together until well blended. Use 1 to 2 tsp. (5-10 mL) per bath.

BATH VINEGARS

The acidity of vinegar serves to counter-act the alkalinity of skin, which in turn makes the vinegar mildly antiseptic and deodorant. In fact, vinegar once held as central a role in the world of skin care as it now does in the culinary arts. Properly made and stored, bath vinegars will last for as long as two years, which is good news if you have a bumper herb crop during the growing season and a surfeit of fresh plant material. Quality dried herbs are almost as effective.

Basic Directions: Place plant material in a glass, ceramic or stainless steel container, and add slightly warmed white or cider vinegar. Cover and leave for several days, shaking or stirring it daily. Strain into a bottle through a fine screen or through several layers of cheesecloth. Be sure to affix a label indicating both the ingredients used and the date the vinegar was made. Add ¼ to 1 cup (50-250 mL) herb vinegar to the bath.

a thoughtful gift, and these oils can also do service as massage oils. You can use a single essential oil or one of the suggested combinations listed below, but before you begin, please see the chapter "Ingredients" and the "Sources" section for information on essential oils. Scented bath oils can also be made without essential oils.

SCENTED BATH OIL FOR DRY SKIN

To ¾ cup (175 mL) sweet almond or olive oil, add ¼ cup (50 mL) avocado oil, 40 drops rose geranium essential oil and 10 drops sandalwood essential oil. Swirl together until well blended. Use 1 to 2 tsp. (5-10 mL) per bath.

SIMPLE BATH VINEGAR

Cover the chopped plant material with slightly warmed vinegar. You can choose from the following herbs, using them individually or in combination: calendula, camomile, lady's mantle, lavender, lemon balm, mints, rose petals, rosemary, sage, scented-geranium leaves or strawberry leaves. Use ¼ to 1 cup (50-250 mL) per bath.

DEODORANT BATH VINEGAR

In 2 cups (500 mL) vinegar, steep a handful or two of one of *or* a combination of: lavender flowers, nettle, parsley, rose petals or thyme. Use ¼ to 1 cup (50-250 mL) per bath.

REFRESHING BATH VINEGAR

In 2 cups (500 mL) vinegar, steep the peel and juice from 1 grapefruit *or* 2 lemons *or* 3 limes. Add a handful of peppermint or other mint and several sprigs of basil. Use ¼ to 1 cup (50-250 mL) per bath.

BATH VINEGAR FOR FATIGUED MUSCLES

In 2 cups (500 mL) vinegar, steep ¼ cup (50 mL) crushed bay leaves, about 20 crushed juniper berries and a bunch of sage leaves, dried or fresh. Use ¼ to 1 cup (50-250 mL) per bath.

BODY SCRUBS

We do our skin an invaluable service when we give it an extra scrub every so often to get rid of stubborn dead cells. Whether it is in the deep of a long, harsh winter or in the middle of an unrelentingly humid summer, removing that extra layer of skin can offer you a refreshing new lease on life. If you have oily skin, I recommend this kind of attention about once a week. For those with normal skin, once or twice a month is sufficient.

Some men and women pay a handsome price to have an attendant at a spa or beauty clinic perform this little act of kindness. But for a few pennies and less time and trouble than it would take to get to a spa, you can make a body scrub part of your regular skin-care ritual in your own home.

Basic Directions: Scrubs should ideally be undertaken while you are standing in a bathtub, since they tend to be somewhat messy. First, have a quick shower or bath to remove any excess sweat or grime from your skin. Then dip a facecloth or loofah pad into your scrub mixture, and slowly work it into your skin in a circular motion, avoiding any open wounds, cracks or irritations. Repeat that motion until you've covered your entire body and the scrub is used up. Remember to go gently. Rinse with warm water, and do not use soap. Pat dry.

SEA-SALT SCRUB

This is an incredibly effective scrub that will leave your skin feeling wonderfully smooth. Once you've rinsed it off, you will still feel a little oily, but that will quickly disappear as the oil is absorbed into your skin. Be sure that the salt is neither too powdery nor too coarse.

¼ cup (50 mL) sea salt or lightly ground pickling salt

Strawberry
Fragaria vesca

¼ cup (50 mL) oil (olive, sweet almond, sunflower, grape-seed or sesame)

2 Tbsp. (30 mL) mild soap-based shampoo *or* 1 tsp. (5 mL) finely grated Castile or glycerin soap moistened with 2 Tbsp. (30 mL) hot water

In a plastic or other nonbreakable container, mix the salt with the oil. Slowly add the shampoo or soap, stirring with your finger. When it's thoroughly mixed, use according to Basic Directions.

YOGURT-BRAN SCRUB

Gentle and refreshing, especially in summer, this scrub is safe for sensitive skin.

½ cup (125 mL) plain yogurt

½ cup (125 mL) wheat bran

2 Tbsp. (30 mL) oil (sunflower, corn or peanut)

2-3 Tbsp. (30-45 mL) apple, pear or cucumber, peeled, seeded and puréed (optional)

Mix yogurt and bran in a nonbreakable container, then thoroughly blend in oil. Add the fruit, if using, and mix well. Use according to Basic Directions.

ALMOND-OATMEAL SCRUB

For dry or sensitive skin begging for a pick-me-up, this scrub is ideal.

2 Tbsp. (30 mL) ground almonds

¼ cup (50 mL) ground rolled oats or oat flour

3 Tbsp. (45 mL) sweet almond or olive oil

¼ cup (50 mL) yogurt

2-3 Tbsp. (30-45 mL) banana or avocado, mashed well (optional)

Lightly grind the almonds and rolled oats or flour in a blender or mortar. In a nonbreakable container, blend the almond mixture with the oil. Add the yogurt and banana or avocado. Mix well. Use according to Basic Directions.

MELON-CORNMEAL SCRUB

This scrub is especially refreshing after a bout of physical labour and for those who are fasting.

½ small, very ripe cantaloupe or honeydew melon *or* 2 or 3 very ripe pears

¼ cup (50 mL) cornmeal

2 Tbsp. (30 mL) sunflower or peanut oil

Remove seeds from melon half. Scoop out the flesh, taking care to retain the juices, and place in a nonbreakable container. (If using pears, remove the seeds and cut off the stem; they do not need to be peeled.) Mash until there are no lumps. Sprinkle the cornmeal over the fruit, then add the oil and blend well. If the mix is watery, add a little flour. Use according to Basic Directions.

TOMATO SCRUB

A very astringent scrub, this recipe is for people with oily or large-pored skin. Pineapple can be used instead of tomatoes.

2 or 3 very ripe red tomatoes, chopped, *or* ½ cup (125 mL) chopped fresh pineapple

½ cup (125 mL) cornmeal

3 Tbsp. (45 mL) olive oil

Mash the tomatoes or pineapple well, or lightly whiz in a blender. If the tomatoes aren't very ripe, heat them slightly in a saucepan or microwave until they're limp. Sprinkle with cornmeal, and drizzle the oil over the mixture. Stir until the consistency is that of a thick sauce. If it is watery, add flour. If it is too thick, add water or cider vinegar. Use according to Basic Directions.

FRUIT-SALAD SCRUB

Here is a great way to make use of leftover fruit that is just beyond its prime.

½ cup (125 mL) mashed strawberries, melon, apples, pears, cucumbers,

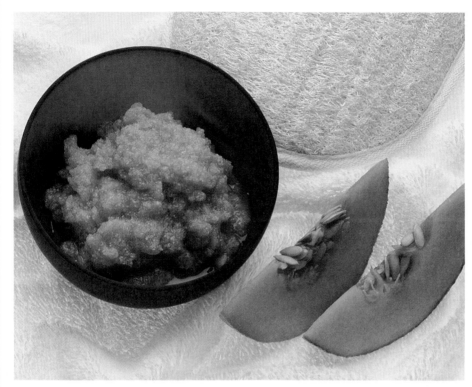

A great summertime melon-based cornmeal scrub.

peaches, bananas, kiwi fruit or avocados *or* a combination of any of these, skinned and seeded where necessary
¼ cup (50 mL) sunflower seeds
2 Tbsp. (30 mL) sesame or sunflower oil
Mash or purée fruit until there are no lumps. In a blender or mortar, grind the sunflower seeds until they are a coarse meal. Add the oil to the seeds, then slowly add the fruit. Stir until smooth, and pour into a nonbreakable container. If the mixture is too watery, add a little flour to thicken. Use according to Basic Directions.

DRY SCRUB

This is a heavy-duty scrub, so be sure to apply it moderately.
1 Tbsp. (15 mL) sea salt or pickling salt
2 tsp. (10 mL) cornmeal
2 tsp. (10 mL) barley
2 tsp. (10 mL) oatmeal
2 tsp. (10 mL) almonds
3 Tbsp. (45 mL) olive oil
Grind dry ingredients together in a blender or mortar until fine. Slowly add the oil, and mix until well blended. Dip a damp cloth into the mix, and work slowly in a circular motion into skin that is slightly moist. When done, lightly rinse off and pat dry.

LIQUID BATH SOAPS

One of the most respected and accessible references for making your own soap continues to be *The Art of Soapmaking* by Merilyn Mohr, also published by Camden House. The recipes that appear here, however, call for the use of store-bought Castile or glycerin soaps. Let

*Refreshing
peppermint and
soothing
camomile liquid
bath soaps.*

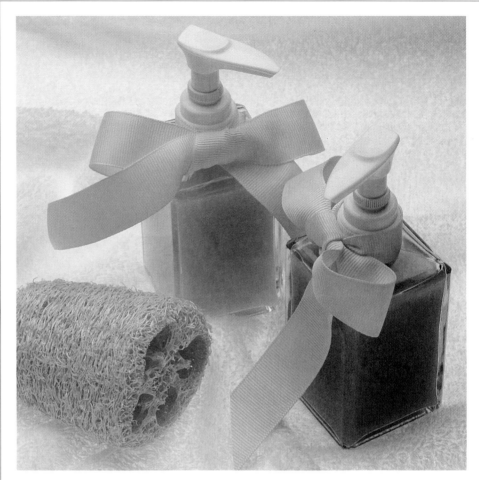

each of these recipes sit for several days before using.

SIMPLE LIQUID BATH SOAP

½ cup (125 mL) shredded glycerin soap
2 cups (500 mL) distilled water
A pinch of borax

Place the soap in a double boiler or a heavy saucepan over low heat. Add the water gradually, stirring gently. Add borax. Keep stirring until the soap has melted. Let cool, then store in a recycled shampoo or liquid-soap bottle. Be sure to label and date the container. For the following recipes, simply replace the distilled water with the described infusion.

HERBAL LIQUID BATH SOAP

Make an infusion, or strong herbal tea, with one of *or* a combination of several of the herbs listed in the following recipes. Using 2 cups (500 mL) of a strong infusion instead of the distilled water, follow the directions as given in Simple Liquid Bath Soap.

REFRESHING LIQUID BATH SOAP

This recipe has a slightly invigorating effect. Make 2 cups (500 mL) of a strong infusion using one of *or* a combination of: peppermint or other mints, basil, rosemary or scented geranium. Then follow the directions as given in Simple Liquid Bath Soap.

SOOTHING LIQUID BATH SOAP

Make 2 cups (500 mL) of a strong infusion using one of *or* a combination of: camomile, rose, lavender or lemon verbena. Then follow the directions as given in Simple Liquid Bath Soap.

LEMON LIQUID BATH SOAP

All these herbs are toning and mildly astringent. To make 2 cups of a strong infusion, use one of *or* a combination of: lemon thyme, lemon verbena, lemon balm, lemon-scented geranium or lemon grass. Then follow the directions as given in Simple Liquid Bath Soap.

SCENTED LIQUID BATH SOAPS

Make the recipe for Simple Liquid Bath Soap. When cooled, add one of the following essential-oil combinations, and shake or stir well. Shake well before using.

LAVENDER LIQUID BATH SOAP

Add 30 drops lavender essential oil to Simple Liquid Bath Soap.

CAMOMILE LIQUID BATH SOAP

Add 15 drops Roman or German camomile essential oil to Simple Liquid Bath Soap.

CITRUS LIQUID BATH SOAP

Add 30 drops mandarin, tangerine or orange essential oil to Simple Liquid Bath Soap.

REFRESHING LIQUID BATH SOAP

Add 20 drops geranium or bergamot orange essential oil to Simple Liquid Bath Soap.

WOODSY LIQUID BATH SOAP

Add 20 drops rosemary, spruce or balsam fir essential oil to Simple Liquid Bath Soap.

*Our bodies are
our gardens, to
which our wills
are gardeners.
—William
Shakespeare,
Othello*

BODY CARE

Our skin breathes for us, cleanses us and registers pain, heat and cold

for us. Although it serves as a kind of shield, protecting us from the

sun and wind and miraculously repairing itself after injury, it also acts

as a two-way conduit, releasing toxins from our bodies and absorbing

the good from the oils, lotions, creams and ointments we smooth onto

it. ❧ Despite the fact that our muscles, tissues and bones are held to-

gether by a common organ—the skin—every part of the body needs

special attention. Sore backs, aching arms, tired feet and dry hands cry

out for a little indulgence. In this chapter, you can choose from a range

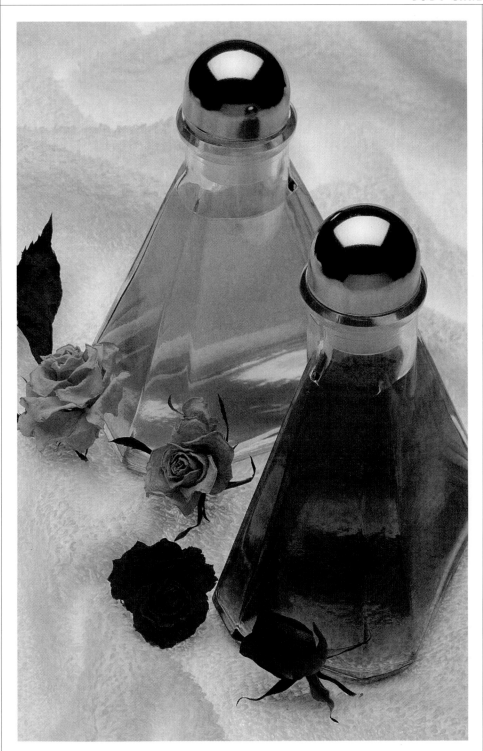

An Invigorating Splash made with peppermint and rosemary as well as a Soothing Splash made with lavender and roses.

of recipes, from those that soothe, relax and console the body to those that will invigorate and inspire.

BODY SPLASHES

When the weather is hot and muggy, I have a secret weapon: a little squeeze bottle containing a vinegar body splash that I use to refresh the back of my neck, arms and legs. The scent of the vinegar dissipates in a few minutes, leaving behind a faint bouquet of herbs. It's a handy travel trick for those times when you'd like to wash up but can't. If you are using a splash after the bath or shower, rub a small amount all over your body while your skin is still moist.

Basic Directions: Follow these directions for each of the body-splash recipes. Place chopped or crushed plant material in a jar or other glass, ceramic or stainless steel container, and cover with slightly warmed white vinegar. Close container, and leave for at least a few days, remembering to shake or stir it daily. Once it is well steeped, strain. I keep the vinegar full strength, labelled, in a glass container. When I am ready to use it, I fill a clean recycled shampoo bottle with one part vinegar and four parts distilled water. Be sure to label this container as well with the date and a description of the herbs used. These splashes should last up to two years. Snap-top caps or spray-pump bottles are handy dispensers.

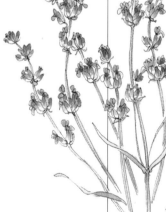

Lavender
*Lavandula
angustifolia*

INVIGORATING SPLASH

This splash is a "wake-up call" if ever there was one.

1 cup (250 mL) white vinegar
1 small bunch fresh peppermint or
  a handful of dried peppermint
1 sprig of fresh rosemary or basil
Peel of 1 lime and half the juice
Once herbs are steeped and strained, add 4 cups (1 L) water. Alternatively, keep full strength, and use in a compress on your forehead when you are experiencing a headache.

SOOTHING SPLASH

If you're prone to heat rashes and other skin irritations, this splash will help. It also has a terrific scent.

1½ cups (375 mL) white vinegar
¼ cup (50 mL) rose- or lemon-scented
  geranium leaves or lavender flowers
¼ cup (50 mL) old-fashioned fragrant
  rose petals *or* replace ¼ cup (50 mL)
  white vinegar with rose water
When steeped and strained, add 4 cups (1 L) water.

DEODORANT SPLASH

Use this splash sparingly, or you may wind up looking as if you've rolled around in a broccoli patch.

1 cup (250 mL) white vinegar
Several dark green lettuce leaves *or* a few
  sprigs of fresh nettles, watercress or
  parsley
A small handful of lavender flowers
Mash or whiz in a blender the lettuce—or nettles, watercress or parsley—with half of the vinegar. Then add the rest of the vinegar and the lavender. Let steep, and strain. Add 4 cups (1 L) water.

SPLASH FOR OILY SKIN

Although intended for oily skin, this splash acts as a toner for all skin types, especially in hot, muggy weather. It is antibacterial, aiding in the control of blemishes.

1 cup (250 mL) white vinegar

¼ cup (50 mL) yarrow leaf and flower or southernwood

1 sprig of fresh rosemary *or* 1 Tbsp. (15 mL) dried rosemary

1 piece of lemon peel

Chop the yarrow or southernwood with the rosemary, then steep with the peel in vinegar. When steeped, strain, and mix with 4 cups (1 L) water.

TONING SPLASH

This splash acts as a toner and a restorative for all skin types. Use half strength as a compress for the eyes.

¾ cup (175 mL) white vinegar

¼ cup (50 mL) witch hazel

2 Tbsp. (30 mL) orange flower water (optional)

¼ cup (50 mL) strawberry leaves, black tea leaves or self-heal

Combine and steep ingredients. Strain, and mix with 4 cups (1 L) water.

SKIN GELS

These gels should be smoothed sparingly all over the body after a bath. They are also effective as a source of quick refreshment.

GEL FOR DRY, SENSITIVE OR MATURE SKIN

In a sturdy pot, gently heat:

¾ cup (175 mL) distilled water

¼ to ½ tsp. (1-2 mL) agar flakes (depending on the desired thickness of the gel)

½ tsp. (2 mL) citric or ascorbic acid

A big pinch of borax

Stir until the dry ingredients are dissolved. Remove from heat, and add:

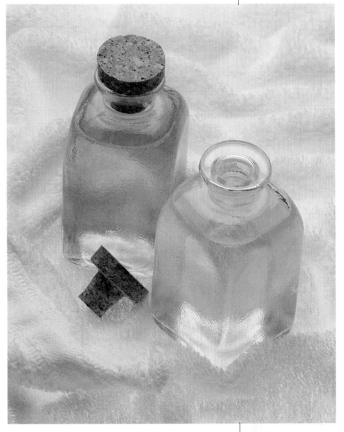

1 Tbsp. (15 mL) rose, orange, lavender or camomile flower water

1 Tbsp. (15 mL) vegetable glycerin or aloe vera gel

1 Tbsp. (15 mL) cider vinegar

1 tsp. (5 mL) tincture or very strong infusion of self-heal, strawberry leaf, marshmallow root, comfrey, slippery elm or camomile

Whisk well, and store in a clean bottle, preferably plastic with a snap-top cap.

GEL FOR NORMAL OR OILY SKIN

In a sturdy pot, gently heat:

¾ cup (175 mL) distilled water

¼ to ½ tsp. (1-2 mL) agar flakes (depending on desired thickness)

A skin gel for dry, sensitive or mature skin and one for normal or oily skin.

Floral-scented body powder to dust on and an unscented body powder to sprinkle on.

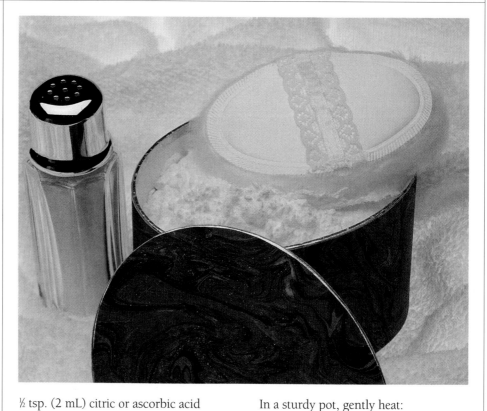

½ tsp. (2 mL) citric or ascorbic acid

A big pinch of borax

Stir until the dry ingredients are dissolved. Remove from heat, and add:

1 Tbsp. (15 mL) witch hazel or rosemary, linden or lavender flower water

1 Tbsp. (15 mL) aloe vera gel

1 Tbsp. (15 mL) cider vinegar

1 tsp. (5 mL) tincture or very strong infusion of nettle, yarrow, echinacea root, wild-carrot seed, red clover, burdock root or white pond lily root

Whisk well, and store in a sterile bottle, preferably plastic with a snap-top cap.

SKIN-SAVIOUR GEL

Soothing and so gentle that it can be safely used on children, this gel is excellent for red, rashy, sunburned or otherwise unhappy skin.

In a sturdy pot, gently heat:

½ cup (125 mL) distilled water

¼ to ½ tsp. (1-2 mL) agar flakes (depending on the desired thickness of the gel)

½ tsp. (2 mL) citric or ascorbic acid

A big pinch of borax

Stir until the dry ingredients are dissolved. Remove from heat, and add:

¼ cup (50 mL) aloe vera gel

1 Tbsp. (15 mL) rose or lavender flower water

1 Tbsp. (15 mL) cider vinegar

1 Tbsp. (15 mL) tincture or very strong infusion of basil, comfrey, marshmallow root, self-heal, black tea, blue violet, chickweed or strawberry leaf

Whisk well, and store in a clean bottle, preferably plastic with a snap-top cap. (For other ways to deal with sunburn, windburn and miscellaneous minor irritations, please see Treatments for Sunburn and Other Skin Crises in the chapter "Kids' Care.")

BODY POWDERS

Sometimes, the stress of everyday living is too much for even the most relaxed among us. Ease the toll taken by anxiety with these simple body-powder recipes.

UNSCENTED BODY POWDER

This is a very plain powder that can be used on the most sensitive skin.

In a container, put:
½ cup (125 mL) cornstarch
To this, add one of *or* a combination of:
1 tsp. (5 mL) orrisroot powder
1 Tbsp. (15 mL) rice flour
1 Tbsp. (15 mL) barley flour
1 tsp. (5 mL) fuller's earth
Mix well, and store powder in a covered container.

FLORAL BODY POWDER

This powder is soothing and has a charming scent.

Use either plain talcum powder or Unscented Body Powder as your base, then carefully add the following, drop by drop:
5 drops lavender or geranium
   essential oil
3 drops petitgrain, bergamot orange
   or orange essential oil
1 drop ylang-ylang, pure jasmine or pure
   rose essential oil
1 drop patchouli or sandalwood
   essential oil
Rub each droplet into the powder with your thumb and forefinger. Mix well, and store in a covered container. Let sit overnight before using to allow the oils to permeate the powder.

WOODSY BODY POWDER

Use either plain talcum powder or Unscented Body Powder as your base, then carefully add the following, drop by drop:
5 drops lemon, lime or grapefruit
   essential oil
3 drops rosemary, balsam fir, spruce or
   juniper essential oil
2 drops frankincense, sandalwood or
   cedar wood essential oil
Rub each droplet into the powder with your thumb and forefinger. Mix well, and store in a covered container. Let sit overnight before using to allow the oils to permeate the powder.

MASSAGE OILS

My idea of a special treat is to make an appointment with a registered massage therapist so that I might relax in the hands of a trained professional. If you can't get to a therapist, you might be lucky enough to have a friend or partner who is willing to give your shoulders a massage when they're stiff. You can also massage your own legs, arms and lower back. These oils will make that experience memorable, whether undertaken in the home or outside it. Lightly rubbed into the skin when it's still moist after a bath or shower, massage oil is as effective as a cream. Many people take their favourite massage oils with them on visits to their massage therapists. Massage oils should be stored in glass bottles and kept in a cool, dark place.

BASIC MASSAGE OIL

This oil is emollient but not too heavy for general massage.

Blend together ½ cup (125 mL) sweet almond oil, ½ cup (125 mL) sunflower, peanut or apricot kernel oil and the contents of 1 capsule of vitamin E.

RICH MASSAGE OIL

To treat very dry skin, combine ¾ cup (175 mL) sweet almond oil, 1 Tbsp. (15 mL) avocado oil, 1 tsp. (5 mL) wheat germ oil, 1 tsp. (5 mL) castor or pure jojoba oil, 1 tsp. (5 mL) infused oil of plantain, mallow leaf, comfrey or camomile and the contents of 1 capsule of vitamin E.

LIGHT MASSAGE OIL

This blend is very light and so is well suited for oily skin or for use in hot, muggy weather. Gently heat ¾ cup (175 mL) peanut or sunflower oil and ¼ cup (50 mL) coconut oil. Remove from heat, and blend in the contents of 1 capsule of vitamin E.

GENTLE MASSAGE OIL

Blend 1 cup (250 mL) of one of *or* a combination of rice bran, apricot kernel or grape-seed oil with the contents of 1 capsule of vitamin E. All these oils have similar consistencies, so you can decide for yourself which proportions you find most pleasing.

AROMATHERAPY MASSAGE OILS

Aromatherapy is a term used to describe the application of aromatic essential oils to the body to achieve a desired effect. For example, a massage oil with lavender not only is very soothing to the nervous system but also helps the skin regenerate. It is important to know which essential oil achieves which effect. Please see the chapter "Ingredients" for the properties of essential oils as well as instructions for handling them.

SIMPLE AROMATHERAPY MASSAGE OIL

A simple aromatherapy massage oil can be made with just one essential oil. Use any of the neutral carrier-oil blends mentioned in the preceding recipes, or use a single oil, such as sweet almond. Please read about diluting essential oils in the chapter "Ingredients." Remember, too, that the scented bath oils which appear in the chapter "The Bath" can also be used as massage oils.

RELAXING MASSAGE OIL

The light floral quality of this oil is soothing and relaxing.

Blend together 1 cup (250 mL) Simple Aromatherapy Massage Oil, 20 drops geranium or lavender essential oil, 12 drops bergamot orange or petitgrain essential oil and 8 drops sandalwood essential oil. Bottle and label.

WARMING MASSAGE OIL

Penetrating and warming, this blend is excellent for chills, chest muscles that have been strained by repeated coughing, bruises and similar complaints. Use sparingly. If you intend to use this blend on bruises, be sure to add the arnica infused oil.

Blend together ½ cup (125 mL) olive or sunflower oil, 20 drops marjoram essential oil, 6 drops frankincense essential oil, 4 drops black pepper essential oil, 20

Marshmallow
Althaea
officinalis

drops arnica infused oil (optional) and the contents of 1 capsule of vitamin E. Bottle and label.

SPORT OIL

Applied either before or after physical exertion, this oil is invigorating and stimulating, especially for the legs and arms. Blend together 1 cup (250 mL) Light Massage Oil, 20 drops rosemary or spruce essential oil, 10 drops lemon or grapefruit essential oil and 5 drops peppermint or camomile essential oil. (You can replace 1 Tbsp. [15 mL] of the Light Massage Oil with infused oil of yarrow, southernwood, St.-John's-wort or ground ivy.) Bottle and label.

DRAWING MASSAGE OIL

This oil is good for oily skin or skin prone to fluid retention.

Blend together 1 cup (250 mL) Light Massage Oil or peanut oil, the contents of 1 capsule of vitamin E, 20 drops lemon or grapefruit essential oil, 14 drops juniper or cypress essential oil and 6 drops camphor or geranium essential oil. (You can replace 1 Tbsp. [15 mL] of the Light Massage Oil with infused oil of yarrow or southernwood.) Bottle and label.

OINTMENTS

Just the sound of the word "ointment" tends to conjure up something horrid-smelling and sticky. Yet the truth is that an ointment is simply a cream without the water, and if it is made with natural ingredients, it does not by definition have to be a thick, gummy paste. An additional benefit is that homemade ointments are easy to make and have a longer shelf life than do creams, which must either contain an antifungal agent or be used quickly. In many instances, soft ointments are every bit as effective for skin care as are creams.

To keep ointments fresh for as long as possible, store in a cool, dark place. The addition of essential oils helps to preserve the ointment and makes it more effective. To help prevent the growth of bacteria, always use a sterile spatula or spoon when removing a portion. If an ointment develops mould or a slightly rancid smell, discard it.

All these recipes call for a bain-marie, or water-bath, and many suggest using an infused oil, so please refer to the chapter "Methods & Equipment" for information about both before you begin. If you want to use petroleum jelly, use slightly less beeswax than the amount called for in the recipe.

BASIC OINTMENTS

Two ointments, soft and firm, act as the base for many creams.

Soft Ointment: A soft ointment is about six parts oil to one part beeswax. In a bain-marie, gently heat ⅓ cup (75 mL) olive oil and 1 Tbsp. (15 mL) pure un-bleached beeswax. When beeswax is melted, remove from heat, and let cool for a few minutes. Stir in the contents of 1 capsule of vitamin E, and pour into a sterile jar. When the ointment has cooled, cover well.

Roman
Camomile
Anthemis nobile

Firm Ointment: About four parts oil to one part beeswax, firm ointment is a stiffer, drier ointment than soft ointment. In a bain-marie, gently heat ¼ cup (50 mL) olive oil and 1 Tbsp. (15 mL) pure unbleached beeswax. When beeswax is melted, remove from heat, and let cool for a few minutes. Stir in the contents of 1 capsule of vitamin E, and pour into a sterile jar. When the ointment has cooled, cover well.

EMOLLIENT OINTMENT

Especially effective for dry or cracked skin, this ointment also soothes minor irritations and protects the skin. In a bain-marie, gently heat 1 Tbsp. (15 mL) pure unbleached beeswax and ⅓ cup (75 mL) infused oil of plantain, camomile, comfrey or mallow leaf. When beeswax is melted, remove from heat, and let cool for a few minutes. Stir in the contents of 1 capsule of vitamin E and 10 drops essential oil of sandalwood, geranium or lavender (optional). Pour into a sterile jar. When the ointment has cooled, cover well.

SKIN-SOOTHING OINTMENT

Any of the following herbs can be used to make cooling and soothing ointments that will also act as skin softeners. In a bain-marie, gently heat 1 Tbsp. (15 mL) pure unbleached beeswax and ¼ cup (50 mL) infused oil of one of *or* a combination of: calendula, blue violet, chickweed, cleavers, comfrey, elder flowers, mallow leaf, plantain or sweet violet. When beeswax is melted, remove from heat, and let cool for a few minutes. Stir in the contents of 1 capsule of vitamin E and 10 drops essential oil of camomile, petitgrain, lavender or geranium *or* 2 drops pure rose essential oil (optional).

Pour into a sterile jar. When the ointment has cooled, cover well.

SUPERMOISTURIZING OINTMENT

This ointment is excellent for very dry skin, especially the hands.

In a bain-marie, gently heat:

1 Tbsp. (15 mL) pure unbleached beeswax

¼ cup (50 mL) olive oil or infused oil of plantain, calendula, mallow leaf, comfrey or camomile

1 tsp. (5 mL) anhydrous lanolin (if you are allergic to lanolin, substitute pure jojoba oil or castor oil)

1 Tbsp. (15 mL) wheat germ, sweet almond or avocado oil

When beeswax is melted, remove from heat, and add:

Contents of 2 capsules vitamin E

Contents of 1 capsule evening primrose oil (optional)

10-20 drops essential oil of sandalwood, lavender, geranium, camomile, bergamot orange, frankincense or ylang-ylang (optional)

Stir well, and pour into one or two sterile jars. Use sparingly.

WARMING OINTMENT

Massage this ointment sparingly into sore muscles, joints and bruises.

In a bain-marie, gently heat:

¼ cup (50 mL) infused oil of comfrey, ground ivy, St.-John's-wort, southernwood or yarrow

1 Tbsp. (15 mL) pure unbleached beeswax

1 tsp. (5 mL) arnica infused oil (optional)

1 tsp. (5 mL) balsam fir gum (optional)

When beeswax is melted, remove from heat, and stir in:

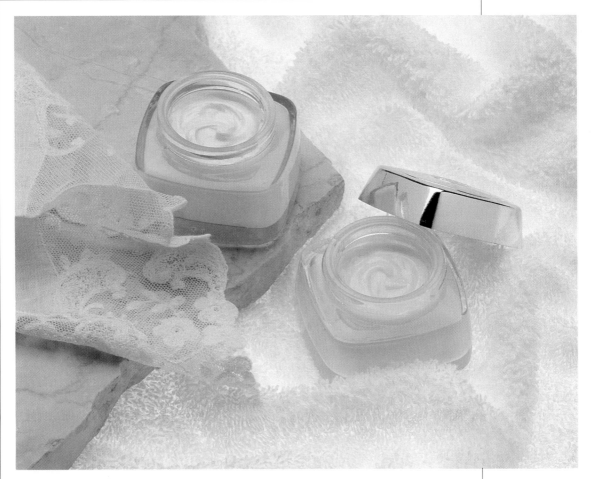

Contents of 1 capsule vitamin E
20 drops tincture of benzoin
10-20 drops essential oil of marjoram,
 eucalyptus, rosemary, camphor, frankincense or spruce *or* 5 drops essential
 oil of cloves
Stir thoroughly, and pour into a sterile
jar. When cooled, cover well.

BALM OF GILEAD OINTMENT
The salicylic acid content of poplar buds
is one of the properties that makes this a
good ointment for sore joints.

In a bain-marie, gently heat ¼ cup (50
mL) infused oil of balm of Gilead (poplar
buds) and 1 Tbsp. (15 mL) pure unbleached beeswax. When beeswax is
melted, remove from heat, and stir in the
contents of 1 capsule of vitamin E, 20
drops tincture of benzoin (optional) and
10 drops essential oil of frankincense,
marjoram or rosemary (optional). Stir
thoroughly, and pour into a sterile jar.
When cooled, cover well.

CREAMS
There are no optional ingredients in
cream; every single one is essential for
the part it plays in the cream's emulsion
and preservation. Creams must be kept
refrigerated, and absolutely sterile uten-

*Avocado and
Orange-Coconut
Creams.*

sils should be used to dispense cream from its container. If the cream develops mould or a rancid smell, it should be discarded.

That said, creams are quite easy to make, once you master the technique. It's much like making mayonnaise.

AVOCADO CREAM

This is a very rich cream that is ideal for dry skin.

In a bain-marie, gently heat ¼ cup (50 mL) avocado oil, 2 tsp. (10 mL) pure unbleached beeswax, 1½ tsp. (7 mL) anhydrous lanolin and 1 tsp. (5 mL) wheat germ oil or infused oil of calendula, St.-John's-wort or plantain. When beeswax is melted, remove from heat.

In a separate pot, gently heat 1 Tbsp. (15 mL) distilled water, 1 tsp. (5 mL) glycerin, a pinch of borax and a pinch of citric acid or a squeeze of strained lemon juice. When dry ingredients are dissolved, remove from heat.

After the oil mixture has cooled for a few minutes, stir in the contents of 1 capsule of soya lecithin. Slowly add half the water mixture to the oil, stirring constantly (you could also use a hand blender on a very low setting). Stir in the contents of 1 capsule of vitamin E. Add the rest of the water slowly, stirring constantly. Then add 10 drops essential oil of patchouli, frankincense, geranium, lavender, sandalwood or ylang-ylang.

When the cream resembles mayonnaise, stop stirring, and pour into a sterile glass jar. (Overstirring can cause the cream to separate.) If cream is still runny, let it cool a minute, stir once more, then pour into jar. When it has cooled completely, cap tightly, label, and store in the refrigerator. Use sparingly.

ORANGE-COCONUT CREAM

This is a lighter cream, more suitable for the face.

In a bain-marie, gently heat until melted ¼ cup (50 mL) coconut oil, 1 tsp. (5 mL) wheat germ oil or calendula infused oil, 2 tsp. (10 mL) pure unbleached beeswax and 1 tsp. (5 mL) anhydrous lanolin. When beeswax is melted, remove from heat.

In a separate pot, gently heat 4 tsp. (20 mL) orange flower water, a pinch of borax and a pinch of citric acid or a squeeze of strained lemon juice. When dry ingredients are dissolved, remove from heat.

After the oil mixture has cooled for a few minutes, stir in the contents of 1 capsule of soya lecithin. Slowly add half the water mixture to the oil, stirring constantly by hand or using a hand blender on a very low setting. Stir in the contents of 1 capsule of vitamin E. Add the rest of the water slowly, stirring constantly. Then add 10 drops essential oil of petitgrain, lavender, bergamot orange or orange *or* 2 drops pure neroli essential oil.

At this point, the cream should resemble mayonnaise. If it does, stop stirring, and pour into a sterile glass jar. Overstirring will cause the emulsion to separate. If the cream is still runny, let it cool a minute, stir once more, then pour into jar. When it has cooled completely, cap tightly, label, and store in the refrigerator. Use sparingly.

BODY SOOTHERS

Whether you're an athlete who's had a rough-and-tumble day on the ball field or tennis court, a gardener who's moved one wheelbarrow of compost too many or someone who's had an accidental fall, these remedies will help soothe your aches and pains.

BRUISE WATER

Use sparingly, by the drop, to treat bruises and strained muscles. Because of the nature of the ingredients, this recipe is not appropriate for children, nor should it be used on broken skin.

To ⅓ cup (75 mL) witch hazel, add 20 drops tincture of arnica, 1 Tbsp. (15 mL) tincture of juniper, rosemary, yarrow or camomile and 20 drops tincture of benzoin. Blend well, and store in a clean plastic or glass bottle that will dispense mixture by the drop. Label bottle.

FRICTION RUB
FOR SORE MUSCLES

Rubbed quickly and lightly onto affected areas, this blend will prove to be refreshing and invigorating.

Coarsely chop one of *or* a combination of camomile, ground ivy, juniper berries, pine needles, rosemary, thyme or yarrow. Place herbs in a glass or stainless steel container, and add a few drops tincture of arnica (optional). Next, add sufficient rubbing alcohol to cover the herbs completely. Put a lid on the container, and let steep for one to two weeks, shaking the mixture every day. Strain, bottle, and label carefully, keeping in mind that rubbing alcohol is poisonous if taken internally.

COOLING RUB

This is a quick pick-me-up on sweltering summer days. It is also a perfect treatment for patients who are confined to bed with a light fever. Cover a quantity of chopped fresh or quality dried peppermint leaves with rubbing alcohol so that the alcohol is twice as deep as the

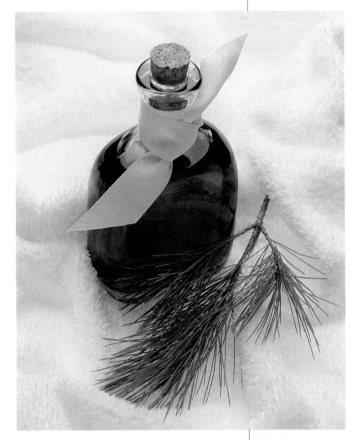

quantity of herbs. Follow the directions given in Friction Rub for Sore Muscles.

FEET AND HANDS

Our feet and hands experience more wear and tear than any other part of our bodies and so demand explicit attention. These recipes have a cosmetic as well as a comfort appeal.

FINGERNAIL SOAK

Before giving yourself a manicure, treat your nails to a soak to help soften the nails and cuticles for grooming. This is also an effective way to fight fungal infections and bacteria that might be lodged around the cuticles and under the nails. The addition of horsetail to a soak will

Pine needles, rosemary and juniper berries make an invigorating friction rub.

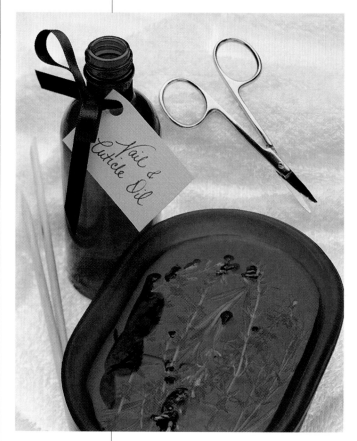

Nail and Cuticle Oil with a Fingernail Soak infused with lavender.

help condition the skin and nails. The other herbs listed here have an antiseptic as well as a conditioning effect.

Make an infusion of one of *or* a combination of: horsetail, calendula, lavender, rosemary, sage or thyme. Soak fingernails for 5 minutes in the infusion when it's tepid. An alternative is to use any of the above herbs in tincture form, adding about ½ to 1 dropperful of tincture to a cup of water.

NAIL AND CUTICLE OIL

To protect and condition the nails, this oil is invaluable. After washing, massage a drop or two into the nails. You need only a couple drops for both hands. This oil can be used on toenails as well.

Mix together:

2 Tbsp. (30 mL) pure jojoba oil

2 Tbsp. (30 mL) sunflower, sweet almond, olive or other vegetable oil or infused oil of calendula or camomile (both antifungal agents), comfrey, mallow leaf or plantain (for very dry skin)

Add:

20 drops essential oil of lavender, rosemary, geranium or eucalyptus

Contents of 1 capsule vitamin E

Blend well, and store the oil in a clean glass bottle.

BURDOCK-SEED INFUSED OIL

Burdock-seed infused oil, either on its own or added to a blend of other oils, is one of the best conditioners for nails. Add a drop or two of vitamin E, and the oil will be more easily assimilated. Use for nails and cuticles.

FOOT SOAK FOR TIRED FEET

In a basin of warm water, add ¼ cup (50 mL) Epsom salts or sea salt and 1 cup (250 mL) infusion of one of *or* a combination of: peppermint, rosemary, thyme, southernwood, pulverized horse chestnut seed, ground ivy or yarrow. (Alternatively, you can use 1 tsp. [5 mL] of any of these herbs in tincture form.) Mix together well, and soak feet for 5 to 20 minutes. After soaking, slip on a pair of cotton socks.

FOOT SOAK FOR ATHLETE'S FOOT

In a basin of warm water, add 1 cup (250 mL) strong infusion of one of *or* a combination of: calendula, thyme, peppermint, sage, lavender or rosemary. (Alternatively, you can use 1 tsp. [5 mL] of any of these herbs in tincture form.) Mix together well, and soak feet for 5 to 10

minutes. Dry feet thoroughly, and dust
between the toes with talcum powder or
cornstarch or with the following recipe
for foot powder.

FOOT POWDER

Refreshing for sore, tired feet, this powder also helps to control the bacteria that
can cause odour or athlete's foot.

In a small container, combine ¼ cup
(50 mL) cornstarch and 1 tsp. (5 mL)
baking soda. Add a pinch or two of orrisroot powder and/or fuller's earth, and
blend well. Add, drop by drop, 2 drops
peppermint essential oil *or* 5 drops rosemary essential oil *or* 5 drops lavender essential oil and an optional drop of thyme
essential oil. Rub the droplets into the
powder between your thumb and forefinger. Mix well, and store in a covered
container. Let sit overnight before using.
A small spice jar with a shaker cap is a
handy dispenser.

FACE CARE

Give me a look,
give me a face,
That makes
simplicity
a grace;
Robes loosely
flowing, hair
as free,
Such sweet
neglect more
taketh me
Than all the
adulteries of art.
—Ben Johnson,
Epicene

On the edge of Mennonite country in southwestern Ontario, where I lived for a couple of years, I often had a chance to visit with these hard-working people as they sold maple syrup and vegetables by the side of the road. While their rough hands and fingernails showed traces of the honest soil in which they had just dug the carrots before them, their faces sported rosy cheeks, shining eyes and reserved smiles. Diets of organically grown produce and meat, plenty of fresh air and a life free of the stresses of urbanization had given them healthy, ruddy complexions. The hard farming life of their convictions had not "ruined" their

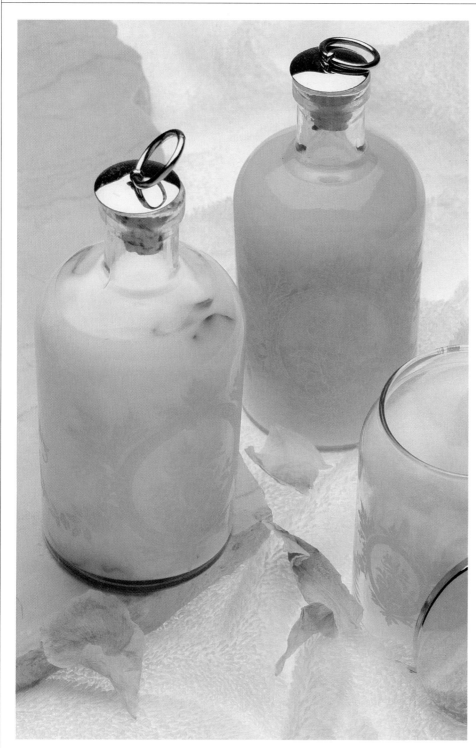

*Rose and
camomile herbal
cleansing
milks can also
be used in
the bath.*

skin; just the opposite: even the elderly had lovely skin. While their life style might not be suitable for many of us, perhaps we can learn from it.

When we meet people for the first time, we look at their faces, their eyes and their mouths and the expressions they choose to reveal. It's almost impossible not to form an impression from these observations, but that's not too surprising. For the face is where we smile, cry, show anger and joy— it's where we tell the stories of our lives. The face is composed of many different muscles, unique in that they are attached to the skin and radiate from the orifices of the face (the mouth, nose and eyes), as well as varying types of skin. The skin around the mouth, for instance, is much stronger and thicker than that around the eyes and, as a result, demands a little specialized attention. The cream you might apply to chapped lips would be the last thing you should use on the delicate skin around your eyes.

With a little care, it is a simple matter to keep the skin on your face healthy, regardless of your age. Remember that smoking, alcohol and caffeine consumption, a poor diet, stress and long-term exposure to central heating or air conditioning can all have detrimental effects

Elder
*Sambucus
canadensis*

on the skin, especially facial skin. If you wear makeup, you have another responsibility—to ensure that it is thoroughly removed at the end of every day. There are also some simple general rules that will stand your face in good stead: Drink lots of water, devise a healthy diet that includes leafy greens and beta-carotene foods, and breathe deeply—it will bring oxygen to your cells. And don't worry about the laugh lines; they tell a story the world needs to hear.

CLEANSERS

The basis of a good complexion is effective cleansing that removes grime, sebaceous secretions, makeup and the like but does not completely strip the skin of its natural oils.

Simple? Yes. But as with most advice, there is a cautionary note: Facial cleansers that claim to clean away *all* oil and grime might be too powerful. If the pores of the skin are dry and taut, secretions cannot escape nor can the skin breathe, and that will exacerbate any skin condition, especially acne. The skin cannot function properly if the pores are closed. You should remember, too, that the body gives off secretions (such as perspiration) even while you sleep, so it's essential to cleanse in the morning as well as at night.

There are many theories on the use of soap for cleansing the face. Some people claim that soap strips the face of its natural oils and leaves it too alkaline; some say that moisturizing soap leaves an unhealthy film on the skin. Others insist that you can't be truly clean unless you use soap. We recommend soaps that contain natural ingredients, such as glycerin or olive oil, because they are gentle and rinse off easily. If you are using hard water, add a few drops of white vinegar or vinegar facial toner to your rinse to help remove any residual film.

There are alternatives to soap, however, and the following recipes will allow you to create cleansers that are both gentle and effective.

YOGURT CLEANSER

For very sensitive skin that is prone to redness or to soothe a hint of sunburn on your face, mix together 1 tsp. (5 mL) plain natural yogurt and 1 tsp. (5 mL) water or herbal infusion (for suggested herbs, see the list that accompanies Herbal Cleansing Milk for Dry or Sensitive Skin).

Gently smooth mixture onto your face, leave for a moment, then rinse with tepid or cool water. You can make up a larger quantity using half yogurt and half water (or a flower water such as rosemary), and store it in the refrigerator. Be sure to use within two weeks.

MAYONNAISE CLEANSER

This cleanser is recommended for dry or mature skin. Smooth 1 to 2 tsp. (5-10 mL) mayonnaise onto your face and throat, wait a moment, then tissue or rinse off. If you are making homemade mayonnaise for this purpose, use lemon juice and a mild oil such as peanut oil, sunflower oil or an inexpensive olive oil along with the egg. If you use commercial mayonnaise, you will notice a lingering "nutty" fragrance, which can be neutralized with a flower water or vinegar toner rinse.

FRUIT CLEANSER FOR OILY OR COMBINATION SKIN

Any of the following fruits are good for cleansing oily and/or large-pored skin: apples, cucumbers, oranges (fresh juice only), peaches, pineapples, strawberries and tomatoes.

Mash well or whiz in a blender or food processor 1 to 2 tsp. (5-10 mL) of one of these fruits. Apply to your face and throat, wait a few seconds, then rinse thoroughly with tepid water. You can juice these fruits and freeze the juice in an ice-cube tray, filling the compartments one-third to one-half full. (You can also freeze the puréed fruit, but add a squeeze of lemon juice to prevent discoloration.) Keep the frozen cubes in a sealed container, and thaw as needed.

FRUIT CLEANSER FOR DRY OR NORMAL SKIN

Apricots, avocados, cucumbers, green or red grapes (not purple), melons, papayas and strawberries are all appropriate fruits for cleansing dry, sensitive or normal skin. To prepare, follow the directions given above (although you might have a little trouble "juicing" an avocado).

CLEANSING MILKS

Milk can be a very gentle cleanser for the face, throat and shoulders, although it loses some of its effectiveness when used on skin that is very soiled or is covered with too much makeup. Milk's lactose, or milk-sugar content, performs a gentle cleansing action when used on the face, as does its butterfat, which has the added benefit of softening or acting as an emollient on your skin. (Soya milk is not a suitable substitute for cow's milk, because it does not have the same composition and is often blended with malt barley, vanilla and other ingredients to make it potable.)

If your skin is dry, the extra butterfat content of whole milk or cream will provide the softening effect you need. For oily skin, use skim milk, which is gentle but has no butterfat content, or buttermilk or diluted yogurt (to dilute, add water until the yogurt has the consistency of milk), both of which, through fermentation, have converted their lactose into lactic acid. That makes them strong yet gentle cleansers.

SIMPLE CLEANSING MILK

Spread 1 to 2 tsp. (5-10 mL) plain milk across your face, using either your fingers or a cotton ball. Leave a moment, then rinse with tepid water. Use whole milk or cream for dry skin and skim milk, buttermilk or diluted yogurt for oily skin.

RICH CLEANSING MILK

This cleanser is for very dry skin.

In a small bottle or bowl, add a few drops of an oil such as wheat germ, sweet almond or olive to 1 to 2 tsp. (5-10 mL) milk. Shake or blend well. For application, use the same directions given in Simple Cleansing Milk.

HERBAL CLEANSING MILK

Take a handful or two of a herb from those listed in Herbal Cleansing Milk for Dry or Sensitive Skin, and steep in 1 cup (250 mL) milk in the refrigerator overnight. Then strain and bottle the milk, and store it in the refrigerator. Because of the nature of this ingredient, you should use it within a few days. You can also freeze the milk in an ice-cube tray, filling the compartments half full. Once frozen, keep the cubes in a sealed container, taking them out one at a time as needed. Herbal Cleansing Milk can also be used in the bath.

HERBAL CLEANSING MILK FOR DRY OR SENSITIVE SKIN

In 1 cup (250 mL) milk, steep overnight in the refrigerator a handful of one of or a combination of the following: ground almonds, borage leaves, calendula flowers, camomile flowers, sweet clover, elder flowers, scented-geranium leaves, lavender flowers, lemon balm, linden flowers, orrisroot pieces, rose petals or sweet violet.

TONING CLEANSING MILK FOR OILY SKIN

In 1 cup (250 mL) buttermilk, steep in the refrigerator overnight a handful of one of or a combination of the following: lavender flowers, lemon thyme, mint, parsley, rosemary, scented-geranium leaves, sage leaves or southernwood leaves. Alternatively, use yogurt, diluted half and half with a tea made from any of these herbs.

GRAIN CLEANSERS

Gently smoothing a grain cleanser onto your face and rinsing it off with a light scrubbing action will remove dead skin cells without damaging the tissue beneath, thus eliminating the need for harsher facial scrubs. Not only are grain cleansers very effective for removing grime, but they leave your skin feeling smooth and revived.

Although these recipes may appear to be slightly more complicated than those we have seen with the other cleansers, they are, in fact, quite simple. I keep a dry mixture of grains in the bathroom in a large jar. That way, it's just a matter of stirring up a little bit at a time in a small bowl. Or, if the oil and water are handy, simply pour a few of the grains into the palm of your hand, add the oil, then the water, mix with your finger, and apply.

GRAIN CLEANSER FOR DRY OR SENSITIVE SKIN

Mix ¾ cup (175 mL) of one of *or* both of:
rice bran flour or finely ground rice
oat bran flour or finely ground oatmeal.
Add 1 Tbsp. (15 mL) comfrey root powder or rose hip powder. Store in a large covered jar or container.

Have on hand ½ cup (125 mL) distilled water or rose, orange or camomile flower water, stored in a glass or plastic bottle, as well as 2 Tbsp. (30 mL) sweet almond oil or Facial Oil for Dry Skin or Facial Oil for Mature Skin. (For facial-oil recipes, see page 79.)

To ½ to 1 tsp. (2-5 mL) grain mixture, add a couple drops of oil, and blend in enough water to make a paste. Smooth onto your face and throat, but do not rub or scrub. Leave on for one minute, then rinse thoroughly with tepid water.

GRAIN CLEANSER FOR NORMAL OR OILY SKIN

Mix ¾ cup (175 mL) of one of *or* both of:
corn flour (not cornmeal)
oat bran flour or finely ground oatmeal
As an option, blend in 1 Tbsp. (15 mL) marshmallow root powder or aloe vera powder. Store in a large covered jar or other container.

Have on hand ½ cup (125 mL) witch hazel, distilled water, lavender or rosemary flower water, stored in a glass or plastic bottle, as well as 2 Tbsp. (30 mL) peanut or sunflower oil or facial oil for oily or normal skin (pages 79-80).

To ½ to 1 tsp. (2-5 mL) grain mixture, add a couple drops of oil, and blend in enough witch hazel or water to make a paste. Smooth onto your face and throat,

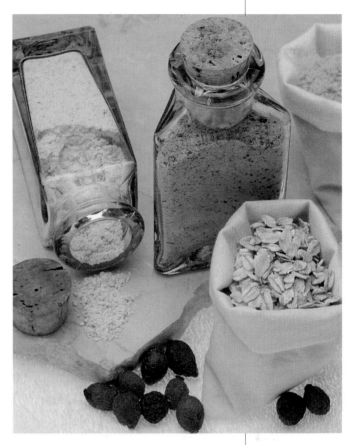

but do not rub or scrub. Leave on for one minute, then rinse thoroughly with tepid water.

TONERS

These days, we hear a lot about muscle tone and how to achieve it through exercise, diet and fresh air. The definition of "tone," according to *Webster's New Collegiate Dictionary*, is "the state of a living body or of any of its organs or parts in which the functions are healthy and performed with due vigor." Since the human body's largest organ is the skin, it shouldn't surprise us that it, too, requires special treatment to perform at its best. And that is where facial toners come in,

Cleansing grains for dry or sensitive skin and for normal or oily skin.

because they have been created to provide the stimulus that will promote good skin health.

Once you've cleansed your face—even if you've used a gentle cleanser—your skin will be at least temporarily bereft of some of its natural barrier, which is composed of secretions. When the skin is "naked" like this, it's an ideal time to apply something that will penetrate the surface to tone, strengthen and balance the sebaceous glands—something astringent for oily skin and something emollient and soothing for dry skin. Many commercial toners contain a lot of alcohol, which dries the skin by contracting the pores unnaturally, thus affecting the skin's ability to breathe and excrete. While some of the toners recommended in this book contain alcohol in the form of tinctures, the amount is small enough that they will not have any adverse effects on the skin.

VINEGAR TONER FOR DRY OR SENSITIVE SKIN

The following herbs are gentle, soothing and emollient and are therefore suited for dry skin.

Take a handful or two of one of or a combination of: borage leaves, calendula flowers, camomile flowers, comfrey root or leaves, lavender flowers, lemon balm, rose petals, scented-geranium leaves, sweet clover or sweet violet. Chop the herbs coarsely, place in a jar, and cover with vinegar (white or cider). Let steep for a week or two, shaking every day. Strain and bottle the liquid.

To use, mix the vinegar with water a bit at a time, one part vinegar to six parts water. You can also use the vinegar as is, a couple drops at a time, to smooth over

your face when it's still moist after cleansing. For very dry skin, add 1 tsp. (5 mL) glycerin for every ½ cup (125 mL) vinegar and water. Glycerin is a humectant, which means that it promotes the retention of moisture.

VINEGAR TONER FOR OILY SKIN

These herbs are astringent and antiseptic. They help draw out secretions without drying the skin, which allows the pores to tighten naturally.

Take a handful or two of one of or a combination of: burdock or yellow dock root, dandelion root, echinacea root, fennel seed, lemon peel, crushed juniper berries, nettle, parsley, rosemary, sage or southernwood. Chop the herbs coarsely, place in a jar, and cover with vinegar (white or cider). Let steep for a week or two, shaking every day. Strain and bottle the liquid.

To use, mix the vinegar with water a bit at a time, one part vinegar to six parts water. As with the toner for dry skin, you can also use the vinegar as is, smoothing a couple drops over your face when it's still moist after cleansing. If you have an acne problem, carry a small bottle of toner with you. You can moisten a tissue or handkerchief with the vinegar to blot up extra facial oil. The vinegar will also help fight bacteria.

VINEGAR TONER FOR NORMAL OR COMBINATION SKIN

These herbs are mildly astringent, emollient and antiseptic and help the skin to function normally.

Take a handful or two of one of or a combination of: calendula flowers, lavender flowers, lemon balm, rosemary, sage or scented-geranium leaves. Chop the herbs coarsely, place in a jar, and cover with vinegar (white or cider). Let steep for a week or two, shaking every day. Strain and bottle the liquid.

To use this toner, mix the vinegar with water a bit at a time, one part vinegar to six parts water.

TINCTURE TONERS

A tincture is a potent concentrated solution that has usually captured a herb at its peak. Its convenience lies in its easy storability (because it is a concentrate, it takes up less space) and its longevity (tinctures keep for years). The vinegar toners listed above can be made as tinctures instead, using the same herbs and the technique described in the chapter "Methods & Equipment."

To use, apply several drops of the tincture to your face when it is moist. Alternatively, mix a bit of the tincture with a few drops of water in the palm of your hand, then apply.

FLOWER-WATER TONERS

Flower waters are excellent toners. Use rose, camomile or orange for dry skin; orange, linden or rosemary for normal skin; and rosemary or witch hazel for oily skin. Lavender can be used for any skin type.

FACIAL OILS

After you've cleansed and toned, a light blend of certain oils will protect your face from the elements while providing other benefits, depending on which blend you choose. Unless your skin is very dry, I recommend using these oils only during the day, since your skin will be healthier if it is allowed to breathe and secrete during the night.

Apply the oil a couple drops at a time, ideally when your face is moist after cleansing. Place one or two drops (depending on the dryness of your skin) on your fingertips, and lightly stroke over your face. Avoid the sensitive skin around your eyes. For a convenient container, use a small eyedropper bottle or a squeeze bottle with a snap top, each of which will hold enough oil to last for several months.

These facial oils can be made without the benefit of essential oils, but what you save in dollars, you will sacrifice in effectiveness and sweet scent.

FACIAL OIL FOR DRY SKIN

This combination of oils is very soothing and emollient and is slightly richer than the others.

2 tsp. (10 mL) peanut oil or sunflower oil

1 tsp. (5 mL) sweet almond oil or olive oil

A few drops of one of *or* a combination of avocado oil, wheat germ oil or calendula infused oil

1 capsule evening primrose oil (optional)

5 drops camomile essential oil *or* 1 drop pure rose essential oil *or* 30 drops camomile infused oil

2 drops ylang-ylang or pure jasmine essential oil

2 drops frankincense or sandalwood essential oil

1 capsule vitamin E

Mix all the oils together, and squeeze in the contents of the vitamin E capsule. Blend well. Makes about 4 tsp. (20 mL).

FACIAL OIL FOR NORMAL OR COMBINATION SKIN

This blend is refreshing and balancing and will help maintain good skin health.

1 Tbsp. (15 mL) peanut oil or sunflower oil

A few drops of one of *or* a combination
of wheat germ oil, calendula infused oil
or St.-John's-wort infused oil

5 drops bergamot orange or petitgrain
essential oil

5 drops lavender or geranium essential
oil

1 capsule vitamin E

Mix all the oils together, and squeeze in
the contents of the vitamin E capsule.
Blend well. Makes about 4 tsp. (20 mL).

FACIAL OIL FOR MATURE SKIN

2 tsp. (10 mL) peanut or sunflower oil

1 tsp. (5 mL) rice bran or apricot
kernel oil

A few drops of wheat germ oil

1 capsule evening primrose oil (optional)

5 drops lavender or petitgrain essential
oil *or* 1 drop pure neroli essential oil

4 drops myrrh or frankincense essential
oil

1 capsule vitamin E

Mix all the oils together, and squeeze in
the contents of the vitamin E capsule.
Blend well. Makes about 4 tsp. (20 mL).

FACIAL OIL FOR OILY SKIN

While this recipe may sound like a contradiction in terms, it works. It helps
draw out the excess oil that causes blemishes, while the essential oils keep bacteria under control.

1 Tbsp. (15 mL) peanut oil

A few drops of one of *or* a combination
of infused oil of yarrow, St.-John's-
wort, rosemary or calendula

3 drops carrot resin oil or beta carotene
(optional)

5 drops lavender or geranium essential
oil

4 drops juniper essential oil *or* 7 drops
lemon essential oil

2 capsules vitamin E

Mix all the oils together, and squeeze in
the contents of the vitamin E capsules.
Blend well. Makes about 4 tsp. (20 mL).

ACNE 'FIRST AID'

For severe cases of acne or a sudden out-
break of blemishes, this blend is effective
in reducing redness and preventing the
spread of bacteria.

Mix an equal amount of lavender essential oil with one of the following essential oils: camphor, cypress, eucalyptus,
geranium or juniper. Store in a small
glass bottle.

To use, dip a cotton swab or other applicator into the oil, and lightly touch
blemishes. Use only once or twice a day.

MISTS

When the skin is dehydrated, it can become unpleasantly dry and taut, which
in turn can lead to the premature formation of wrinkles, especially for people
with thin or dry skin. Healthy skin is
moist enough to allow the various layers
to breathe and function normally. Air
travel, air conditioning, centrally heated
buildings, the wind and the sun are all
part of what sometimes seems to be a
worldwide conspiracy to dry our skin.
But I have discovered an excellent de-
fensive weapon in this ongoing battle:
the mister.

A friend taught me to stash a sturdy
spray-pump bottle, like the one used to
spray plants, in the glove compartment
of my car. When you're stuck in the
middle of a traffic jam on one of the hot-
test, muggiest days of the summer, a
quick spray instantly refreshes. You can

mist with plain water or with one of the blends suggested here. The addition of vinegar to the recipe will help keep your skin fresh and will also control bacteria.

MIST FOR DRY SKIN

Mix together ¾ cup (175 mL) distilled water (you can substitute 1 Tbsp./ 15 mL water with cider vinegar), ¼ cup (50 mL) rose, camomile or orange flower water and a few drops of tincture of comfrey, mallow, plantain, camomile, lavender or geranium. Add a pinch of citric acid or a small squeeze of lemon juice. Store in a spray-pump bottle.

MIST FOR NORMAL OR COMBINATION SKIN

Mix together ¾ cup (175 mL) distilled water (you can substitute 1 Tbsp./ 15 mL water with cider vinegar), ¼ cup (50 mL) lavender, rosemary or linden flower water and a few drops of tincture of lemon balm, rosemary, sage, geranium, calendula or sweet clover. Add a pinch of citric acid or a small squeeze of lemon juice. Store in a spray-pump bottle.

MIST FOR OILY SKIN

Mix together ¾ cup (175 mL) distilled water (you can substitute 1 Tbsp./ 15 mL water with cider vinegar), ¼ cup (50 mL) lavender, rosemary or witch hazel flower water and a few drops of tincture of echinacea, burdock, yellow dock, yarrow, southernwood or juniper. Add a pinch of citric acid or a small squeeze of lemon juice. Store in a spray-pump bottle.

MASKS

Masks that are made of powdered clay, grains or egg whites are an extremely effective way to free the skin of impurities that have been missed by conventional washing. As the mask dries, oils and other pore-clogging matter are gently drawn out, thus helping the pores to function normally. Emollient masks (made with ingredients such as egg yolk) have the opposite effect, allowing emollient and humectant substances to moisturize the skin.

SIMPLE CLAY MASK

Toning and refreshing for normal, combination and oily skins, the clay mask can be used on dry or sensitive skin as well provided that you add a drop or two of facial or other oil to make the mask's effect a little less intense.

Mix 2 tsp. (10 mL) fuller's earth (or other cosmetic clay) with enough water to make a spreadable paste. Smooth the paste onto your face and neck, avoiding the eye area. For dry skin, leave on only five minutes; otherwise, let dry, then rinse with tepid water. If you have oily skin, leave on not only until the mask is dry but until you can see the oil being drawn out from such problem areas as around the nostrils, the chin, and so on.

REFRESHING CLAY MASK

For skin that could use a little enlivening, this mask will do the trick.

To 2 tsp. (10 mL) fuller's earth, add ½ tsp. (2 mL) powdered peppermint leaves and enough water or very strong peppermint tea to make a paste. Smooth the paste onto your face and neck. Leave on

Calendula
Calendula officinalis

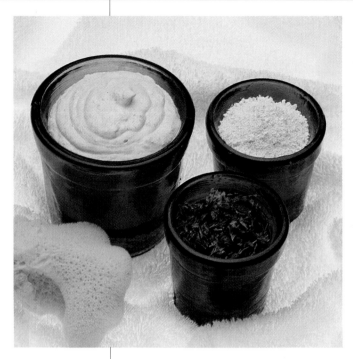

Cooling peppermint clay mask.

for 5 to 10 minutes, then rinse well with tepid water.

HONEY-OATMEAL MASK

This mask acts as a humectant, drawing moisture in. It is terrific for dry or mature skin.

To 2 Tbsp. (30 mL) oat flour or finely ground rolled oats, add enough water or rose water to make a very thick paste. Add 1 tsp. (5 mL) liquid honey. Blend mixture well, and smooth onto face and throat, avoiding the eye area. Leave on for 5 to 15 minutes, then rinse well with tepid water.

EMOLLIENT MASK

This mask is intended for extra-dry skin that is crying out for help.

Place one egg yolk in a bowl, and whisk in 1 tsp. (5 mL) liquid honey. Add a pinch or two of oat flour until the mixture is not quite so runny. Smooth onto your face and throat. Leave on for 5 to

10 minutes, then rinse thoroughly with tepid water.

EGG-WHITE MASK

The binding action of egg white is effective for toning oily and/or large-pored skin. When the mask begins to dry, the egg, flour and clay help to draw out impurities and excess oil.

Whisk a few drops of lemon juice or white vinegar into an egg white. Blend in a pinch or two of oat flour, rice flour and fuller's earth. Smooth thinly onto your face and throat. Leave on for at least 15 minutes before rinsing thoroughly with tepid water.

EYE AND LIP CARE

Last but not least, we have a few recipes for the eyes and the mouth. Obviously, the needs of each are significantly different and require separate treatment, but both are vulnerable to the effects of sun and wind and deserve their own cosmetic pampering.

HERBAL EYE FRESHENER

Take a quantity of one of *or* a combination of: camomile flowers, elder flowers, English daisy, eyebright, fennel seed, marshmallow root, crushed rose hips, rose petals, strawberry leaves or white pond lily root. Cover with enough boiling water to make a strong brew. (You can mix a small quantity of "tea" to use as you need it or make a larger amount. If you do prepare a larger amount, you must either refrigerate it and use within a few days or freeze it in ice-cube trays, filling the compartments half full, then storing the cubes in a covered container and thawing as needed.) Let mixture steep until cool, then strain well so that there are no bits left in the water. For a subtle twist and a soothing effect, add a few drops of rose or orange flower water at this point. For very dry skin, add 1 tsp. (5 mL) glycerin for every ½ cup (125 mL) of brew. If you are making a larger quantity, you must add a preservative: ¼ tsp. (1 mL) citric acid or a healthy squeeze of strained lemon juice for every ½ cup (125 mL) of brew.

To use, close your eyes and gently pat the eye area with the solution, using your fingertips or a cotton ball. To make a soothing compress, soak two cotton balls or pieces of cotton in the solution, and place them over your closed eyes for a few minutes.

Please Note: You can also use any of these herbs in tincture form, but be sure to dilute one part tincture to at least four parts water. And remember: Tinctures contain a small amount of alcohol, and when alcohol comes in contact with the eyes, it stings, so be extra careful!

EYE GEL

Using any of the herbs mentioned in Herbal Eye Freshener, make a strong brew, and strain thoroughly. To ¼ cup (50 mL) infusion, add two big pinches of agar flakes and a small pinch of borax. Gently heat and stir until the agar and borax are melted. Then add a big pinch of citric or ascorbic acid or a small squeeze of strained lemon juice. For eyes that are sore, tired or red, add a few drops of rose water. For dry skin, add a few drops of glycerin.

Whisk together, and pour into a sterile jar with a tight-fitting lid. Store in the refrigerator. Use a cotton swab or other applicator to remove the gel from the jar. (If the gel develops an odour or if mould forms on it, discard.)

Dab lightly around the eyes, but remember to use sparingly.

FLOWER EYE FRESHENERS

Rose, orange and camomile flower water are excellent eye fresheners when diluted by half with water.

LIP CREAM

This is a light ointment that, when used sparingly, will not clog the pores around the mouth. If you have chapped lips or need additional protection for outdoor activities, add a bit of anhydrous lanolin to provide extra emollience.

In a bain-marie, melt together 1 Tbsp. (15 mL) coconut oil, 2 Tbsp. (30 mL) sweet almond or sunflower oil, 2 tsp. (10 mL) pure unbleached beeswax and ¼ tsp. (1 mL) anhydrous lanolin (optional).

When all ingredients have melted, remove double boiler from heat. Let stand a couple minutes, then stir in the contents of 1 capsule of vitamin E. You could also add 5 drops essential oil of sandalwood, myrrh or sage *or* 10 drops tincture of myrrh.

Pour into small, clean jars. Makes about ¼ cup (50 mL).

English Daisy
Bellis perennis

*Fair tresses
man's imperial
race ensnare,
And beauty
draws us with a
single hair.*
—Alexander
Pope, *The Rape
of the Lock*

HAIR CARE

There is no getting around it: Humans are plagued and blessed—and

everything in between—by their hair. Our society places great emphasis

on hair, as an evening's worth of television commercials will quickly

reveal. Is it the right style? Is it the right colour? Is it shiny enough? Is it

clean enough? Is it wavy enough? Is it straight enough? It sometimes

seems as though our success in the world may rise or fall on how we

manage our hair and scalps. My teenage son spends more time in front

of the mirror dealing with his half-inch-length hair than I do with my

considerably longer hair style, but that's because I've lived long enough

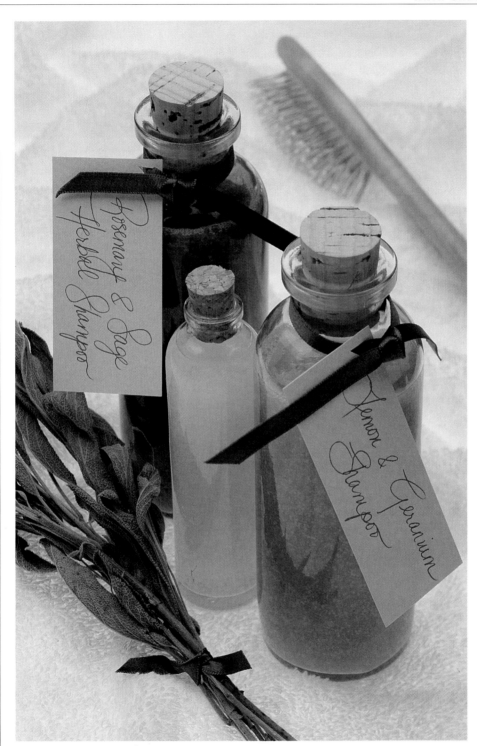

Rosemary and sage herbal shampoo, lemon and geranium aromatherapy shampoo and a small bottle of Basic Glycerin Shampoo.

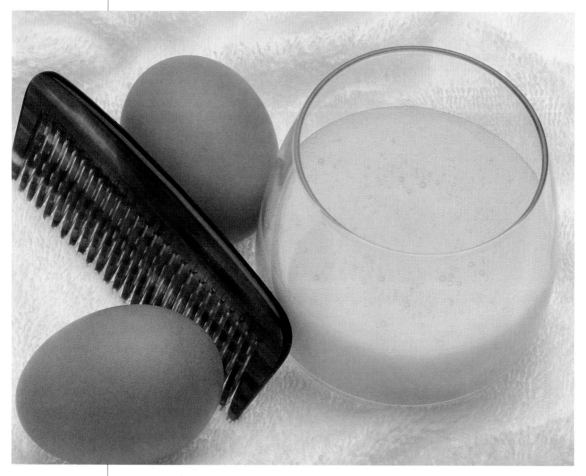

Egg Treatment for Very Dry Hair or Scalp.

to know that whatever its state, I shouldn't let my hair ruin my day. Nevertheless, like most people, I'm always happier when my hair and scalp feel healthy and clean, and the following recipes will address at least that part of the trauma. I'll leave the rest to you.

PRESHAMPOO TREATMENTS

Treating the hair *before* washing can actually help certain scalp and hair conditions. While hair is basically a "dead" extrusion from the body, it is porous in varying degrees. As a result, preshampoo treatments can serve to fill in the overlapping scalelike cells of the hair and give it shine and body.

Most of these recipes list two quantities for some ingredients. If your hair is very short or very fine, use the lesser amount. If your hair is long or very thick, use the greater amount.

After applying the treatment, spread it thoroughly and evenly through your hair with a large-toothed comb.

SIMPLE HOT-OIL HAIR TREATMENTS

Hot-oil treatments are both simple and immediately effective. If you have very dry or fine hair, apply the oil when your hair is dry. If you have very thick, long or curly hair, moisten it slightly so that the oil will be distributed evenly.

Basic Directions: In a stainless steel pot, gently heat 1 to 2 Tbsp. (15-30 mL) oil until it is comfortably warm to the touch. Dip your fingertips into the oil, and begin to work it into the hair, starting at the scalp. Use a large-toothed comb to distribute it evenly through the hair. When all the oil has been applied, cover hair with plastic wrap or wax paper, then wrap head with a warm towel. Leave on for 5 to 30 minutes. Before you wash your hair, apply a bit of shampoo directly to the hair first to emulsify with the oil. Then add water, and shampoo as usual. Rinse, and repeat.

Don't be afraid to combine oils. If you have dry, dark hair, you can blend olive oil with a bit of avocado oil, for example. To create a personalized treatment, choose one of *or* a combination of any of the following oils, based on your hair type.

For Fair Hair: calendula infused oil, camomile infused oil, peanut oil, rice bran oil or sunflower oil

For Dark Hair: olive oil, rosemary infused oil or St.-John's-wort infused oil

For Dry Hair or Scalp: avocado oil, comfrey infused oil, pure jojoba oil, mallow-leaf infused oil, plantain infused oil, sweet almond oil or wheat germ oil

EGG TREATMENT FOR VERY DRY HAIR OR SCALP

While you nourish your hair with the egg yolk, give yourself a pore-tightening facial with egg white and lemon (see page 82).

In a bowl, whisk together one or two egg yolks. As you whisk, add a few drops of lemon juice or white vinegar, then blend in 1 to 2 Tbsp. (15-30 mL) avocado, wheat germ or olive oil. When your "mayonnaise" is emulsified, smooth through hair with a large-toothed comb or massage into scalp. Cover head with plastic wrap or wax paper, then wrap with a towel, and leave on for 5 to 30 minutes. To shampoo, massage a little shampoo directly into the hair first before adding water. Slowly add tepid, not hot, water, then shampoo, rinse, and repeat. Follow with a white-vinegar- or lemon-juice-based rinse.

MAYONNAISE TREATMENT FOR DRY HAIR OR SCALP

Commercial or homemade mayonnaise can be used as a preshampoo treatment for dry hair or scalp. Thin the mayonnaise slightly by whisking in a little lemon juice or white vinegar, then use as you would the egg treatment.

HONEY TREATMENT FOR DRY HAIR OR SCALP

Place a small bowl in a larger bowl half filled with hot water. In the small bowl, combine 1 to 2 tsp. (5-10 mL) liquid honey and 1 to 2 Tbsp. (15-30 mL) olive oil or infused oil of calendula, camomile, plantain, mallow leaf or comfrey. When

St.-John's-Wort
Hypericum perforatum

the honey and oil are melted together, apply mixture to lightly dampened hair or scalp. Cover with plastic wrap or wax paper. Wrap head with a warm towel, and leave on for 5 to 30 minutes. Massage a little shampoo directly into hair first before adding water. Shampoo, rinse, and repeat. Follow with a white-vinegar- or lemon-juice-based rinse.

SHAMPOOS

Many commercial shampoos now contain natural ingredients, so we are under a little less pressure to create our own. Shampoos with coconut- and palm-oil bases seem to have taken the lead in the popularity contest, and the good news is that they are not only effective but biodegradable as well. Alternatively, I have a friend who regularly uses a mild glycerin or Castile bar soap on his hair. The only drawback is that bar soaps tend to leave a dull film on the hair shaft. That can be remedied, however, with a white-vinegar- or lemon-juice-based rinse, which will remove the film and leave a lustrous shine.

The recipes that follow are for mild shampoos which do not produce a lot of lather. These shampoos are especially recommended for people with sensitive skin. Be sure to follow with a white-vinegar- or lemon-juice-based rinse. Let all of these shampoos sit for a few days before using.

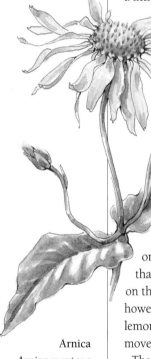

Arnica
Arnica montana

BASIC CASTILE SOAP SHAMPOO

In a bain-marie, place ½ cup (125 mL) grated Castile soap. Add 1 Tbsp. (15 mL) coconut oil and a pinch of borax. (For dry hair, you can also add ½ tsp. (2 mL) avocado, sweet almond or wheat germ oil.) When coconut oil has blended with melted soap, slowly add 2 cups (500 mL) distilled water. Stir constantly until the water is incorporated with the soap. Bottle and label.

BASIC GLYCERIN SHAMPOO

In a bain-marie, place ¼ to ⅓ cup (50-75 mL) grated glycerin soap. Add a pinch of borax. Slowly add 2 cups (500 mL) distilled water. Stir constantly until the water is incorporated with the soap. Bottle and label.

HERBAL SHAMPOOS

Instead of adding distilled water to Basic Castile Soap Shampoo or Basic Glycerin Shampoo, substitute an infusion made with any of the herbs listed under "Rinses" (see next page).

AROMATHERAPY SHAMPOOS

To create an aromatherapy shampoo, simply add essential oils to Basic Castile Soap Shampoo or Basic Glycerin Shampoo. Because of the volatility of essential oils, wait until the shampoo has cooled completely before adding them. (You can also add essential oils to unscented or very mildly scented store-bought shampoos.) Put a spoonful or two of shampoo in a small bowl. Mix in the oils, then blend back into the larger amount. These recipes are for 2 cups (500 mL) shampoo, so adjust the amount of essential oil you use accordingly.

AROMATHERAPY SHAMPOO FOR FAIR HAIR

For 2 cups (500 mL) shampoo, add 20 drops lemon essential oil and 10 drops camomile essential oil.

AROMATHERAPY SHAMPOO FOR DARK HAIR

For 2 cups (500 mL) shampoo, add 15 drops rosemary essential oil and 5 drops patchouli essential oil.

AROMATHERAPY SHAMPOO FOR OILY HAIR

For 2 cups (500 mL) shampoo, add 20 drops essential oil of lemon, lime, grapefruit, tangerine or orange and 5 drops juniper or cypress essential oil.

AROMATHERAPY SHAMPOO FOR DRY HAIR

For 2 cups (500 mL) shampoo, add 15 drops camomile or geranium essential oil, 5 drops cedar wood or sandalwood essential oil and 1 tsp. (5 mL) avocado oil (optional).

AROMATHERAPY SHAMPOO FOR PROBLEM SCALPS

For 2 cups (500 mL) shampoo, add 20 drops eucalyptus or lavender essential oil, 1 drop thyme essential oil (optional) and a few drops arnica infused oil or tincture (optional).

RINSES

These rinses are not a solution for tangled hair, but they have other benefits. Herbal rinses not only refresh the scalp and alleviate oily or dry-hair conditions but can add lustre to dark hair and sparkle to fair.

Basic Directions: Using the herbs suggested for your hair type, you can make rinses in a variety of ways. If you have hard water or use a bar soap to wash

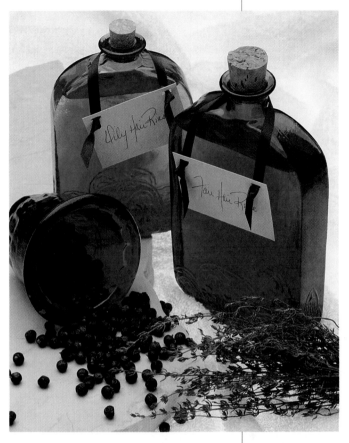

your hair, a white-vinegar- or lemon-juice-based rinse worked thoroughly through your wet hair will help to counter the alkalinity and remove any soap residue. If the residue seems to linger, simply rinse again. Otherwise, you should apply the rinse once, and leave it on your hair.

Herbs for Dry or Fine Hair Rinse: Use one of *or* a combination of the following emollient herbs: Roman camomile, comfrey root, horsetail, marshmallow root, plantain or scented geranium.

Herbs for Oily Hair Rinse: Use one of *or* a combination of: bay leaf, juniper berries, nettle, southernwood or yarrow.

Herbs for Dark Hair Rinse: Use one of *or*

Herbal rinses to refresh the scalp.

a combination of: black tea (1 tsp. [5 mL] per cup), lavender, rosemary or sage.

Herbs for Fair Hair Rinse: Use one of *or* a combination of: calendula, camomile, lemon peel or scented geranium.

Herbs for Problem Scalp Rinse: Use one of *or* a combination of: bay leaf, birch (either leaves or bark), burdock seed, comfrey root, juniper, lavender, nettle, sage or thyme.

INFUSION

Make a mild infusion using 1 Tbsp. (15 mL) herb to 1 cup (250 mL) water. When the infusion has cooled, strain off the herbs, and pour the remaining liquid over wet hair after washing.

TINCTURE RINSE

Use a single or combination tincture of any of the herbs listed below, adding ½ to 1 tsp. (2-5 mL) tincture to 1 cup (250 mL) water.

LEMON JUICE RINSE

Add the strained juice of half a lemon or ¼ tsp. (1 mL) citric acid to 1 cup (250 mL) infusion. The lemon will add sparkle to fair hair.

VINEGAR RINSE

Chop one or two handfuls of herbs, place in a container, and cover with white vinegar. Seal the container, and let steep for a week, shaking it every day. Strain, and keep until needed. Mix one part vinegar to four parts water, and pour over wet hair after washing.

OILS

If you use pure jojoba oil in either of the following recipes, your hair will actually feel "dry," rather than greasy. Oil can refresh the scalp and add lustre to the hair shaft. Simply place one or two drops in the palm of your hand, and rub the ends of your hairbrush bristles in it. Brush through your hair until the oil is evenly distributed. Men can also use oil on their beards. Burdock-seed infused oil is a good hair conditioner and an effective dandruff treatment.

OIL FOR FAIR HAIR

Mix together 2 Tbsp. (30 mL) pure jojoba or castor oil, 2 Tbsp. (30 mL) sunflower or peanut oil or infused oil of calendula or camomile, 20 drops essential oil of camomile, lemon or geranium and a few drops of burdock-seed infused oil (optional). Squeeze in the contents of 1 capsule of vitamin E. Blend well, and store in a clean bottle.

OIL FOR DARK HAIR

Mix together 2 Tbsp. (30 mL) pure jojoba or castor oil, 2 Tbsp. (30 mL) sunflower or olive oil or infused oil of St.-John's-wort or rosemary, 20 drops essential oil of lavender, rosemary or patchouli and a few drops burdock-seed infused oil (optional). Squeeze in the contents of 1 capsule of vitamin E. Blend well, and store in a clean bottle.

HAIR AND SCALP CONDITIONERS

Here are two easy-to-make conditioners—one for the hair and one for the scalp—that will make both healthier.

FLOWER-GLYCERIN DRESSING

A very simple recipe that will give your hair great body.

Blend together ½ cup (125 mL) flower water, 1 Tbsp. (15 mL) glycerin and a pinch of borax. Stir until the borax dissolves. Bottle and label. To use, rub several drops into your hair. Can be used on damp or dry hair. Comb through.

SCALP TONIC

For those with dry scalps who suffer from dandruff as a result.

Blend together ⅓ cup (75 mL) distilled water (you can substitute 2 Tbsp. [30 mL] of the distilled water with rosemary or camomile flower water), 2 Tbsp. (30 mL) white vinegar, a pinch of borax and ½ tsp. (2 mL) tincture of one of *or* a combination of burdock seed, burdock root, yellow dock root, echinacea, arnica, nettle, juniper, comfrey, marshmallow, lavender, sage or thyme. Mix until borax dissolves. Bottle and label. To use, rub a few drops directly onto the scalp, then comb through.

KIDS' CARE

Smooth, soft and sweet-smelling, children's skin has an innocence about it that almost defies description. In an ideal world, where we could guarantee our young perfect care and protection, that condition might extend until adolescence, when the skin stages its own rebellion. But for those fleeting early years, the skin of our children cries out for tender treatment. Perhaps that is why it is so unsettling to us when something mars its unblemished surface. ❧ The reality is that children's bodies change so rapidly, we can often count on them simply to outgrow certain complaints. A balanced, nutritious diet and regular

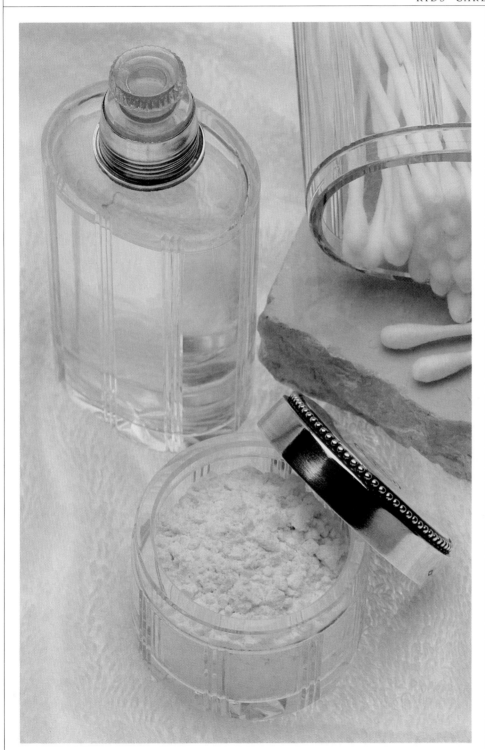

*Baby Powder
and rich Baby
Oil for tender
young skin.*

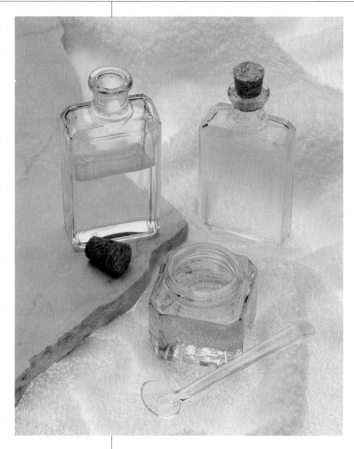

Honey-Flower Lotion made with honey and orange flower water.

skin, and leave it there overnight to see whether there is any reaction.

These recipes are also suited to adults who have sensitive skin.

BABY OIL

This is a lovely rich oil that can be used not only for babies still in diapers but for children with dry skin and as a massage oil. If your child suffers from very dry skin or diaper rash, replace the sunflower oil with sweet almond oil.

⅓ cup (75 mL) sunflower, rice bran, apricot kernel or grape-seed oil
⅓ cup (75 mL) sweet almond oil
2 Tbsp. (30 mL) olive oil or infused oil of calendula, camomile, mallow leaf or plantain
1 tsp. (5 mL) wheat germ oil
6 drops lavender essential oil *or* 2 drops camomile essential oil *or* 1 drop pure rose essential oil (optional)
1 capsule vitamin E

Blend ingredients together, squeezing in the contents of the vitamin E capsule. Label and store in a plastic squeeze bottle.

BARRIER OINTMENT

Desperate times call for desperate measures, and when your child is suffering from a serious diaper rash, it's time to deploy a thick barrier ointment. (Please refer to the chapter "Body Care" for more information about ointments.)

In a bain-marie, gently heat 2 Tbsp. (30 mL) pure unbleached beeswax with ½ cup (125 mL) olive oil, sweet almond oil or infused oil of calendula, comfrey, plantain or marshmallow root. When the beeswax has melted, remove from heat. Stir in the contents of 2 capsules of vitamin E and 5 drops lavender essential oil (optional). Pour into a sterile jar with a tight-fitting lid. For best storage, keep in

bathing goes a long way to ensuring that your child has healthy skin. Nevertheless, occasional problems—diaper rash and sunburn are two—can make your child so uncomfortable that immediate and thoughtful attention is required. For minor problems such as these and for straightforward skin care, I offer a few simple recipes, with the counsel that a professional should be consulted for more serious or ongoing difficulties.

If you are concerned that your child might have sensitivities to any of the herbs or oils contained in these recipes, you can perform a simple patch test before using: Dab a little bit of the substance on a small area of your child's the refrigerator or a cool place. Use a clean spatula or cotton swab when removing from the jar.

HONEY OINTMENT

Ideal for children with dry skin, this ointment is also an effective moisturizer to guard against the elements.

In a bain-marie, gently heat ½ cup (125 mL) sweet almond oil, 2 Tbsp. (30 mL) pure unbleached beeswax and 1 Tbsp. (15 mL) liquid honey. When melted, remove from heat. Add the contents of 1 capsule of soya lecithin and 1 capsule of vitamin E and 5 drops camomile or geranium essential oil (optional). Stir well, and pour into a sterile jar with a tight-fitting lid. Use a clean spatula or cotton swab when removing from the jar.

HERBAL OINTMENTS

Using the recipe described on page 65 in the chapter "Body Care," make a soft ointment of six parts oil to one part pure unbleached beeswax, using any of the following infused oils: calendula, camomile, marshmallow root, plantain, chickweed, cleavers or sweet violet, all of which are suitable for children. To find out the benefits of each herb, refer to the chapter "Ingredients."

MALLOW-ROSE CREAM

Remember that there are no optional ingredients for cream; every single one is essential to the emulsion, so do not attempt any shortcuts. Mallow-Rose Cream, a soothing emollient that is good for both children and adults, is based on a recipe created almost 2,000 years ago by Galen, a Greek physician who was the father of all cosmetic emulsions.

In a bain-marie, gently heat until all has melted:

¼ cup (50 mL) sweet almond oil or

infused oil of marshmallow root or comfrey root

1 tsp. (5 mL) sweet almond oil or infused oil of calendula, blue violet, chickweed or plantain

2 tsp. (10 mL) pure unbleached beeswax

1½ tsp. (7 mL) anhydrous lanolin

In a separate pot, gently heat until the dry ingredients have dissolved:

4 tsp. (20 mL) rose water

A pinch of citric acid or a squeeze of strained lemon juice

A pinch of borax

Remove both pots from the heat. Allow oil mixture to cool for a few minutes, then stir in the contents of 1 capsule of soya lecithin. Slowly add half the water mixture to the oil, stirring constantly (or use a hand blender on a very low setting), then add the contents of 1 capsule of vitamin E. Slowly add the rest of the water, stirring constantly. Then add 10 drops essential oil of camomile, lavender, geranium, sandalwood, myrrh, ylang-ylang or petitgrain.

At this point, the cream should have the consistency of mayonnaise. If it does, stop stirring, and pour into a sterile glass jar. Overstirring can cause the emulsion to separate. If it is still runny, let it cool a minute, stir once again, then pour into a jar. When it has completely cooled, cap tightly and store in the refrigerator. Re-

Sweet Violet
Viola odorata

A herbal bath tea of red clover and rose petals can be added to bathwater to treat mild skin complaints.

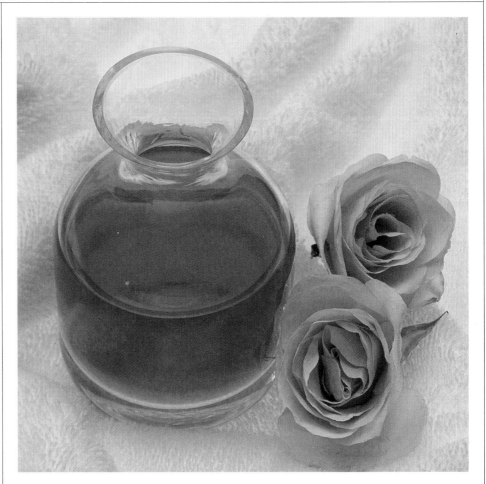

move from jar with a clean utensil, and use sparingly.

HONEY-FLOWER LOTION

A pleasant lotion that will lightly moisturize and soothe red or irritated skin, Honey-Flower Lotion may seem a bit sticky when you first rub it onto the skin. After a few minutes, however, that sensation will disappear.

In a saucepan, lightly warm ¼ cup (50 mL) distilled water, 1 tsp. (5 mL) liquid honey and ¼ tsp. (1 mL) citric acid. When the honey is dissolved, remove from heat, and stir in 2 Tbsp. (30 mL) flower water (lavender, rose, orange or camomile) and 2 Tbsp. (30 mL) glycerin. Pour into a clean bottle, and label.

BABY POWDER

In a bowl, blend ⅓ cup (75 mL) cornstarch, 2 Tbsp. (30 mL) rice flour, rice bran flour or oat flour and an optional pinch of marshmallow root powder.

Add 5 drops lavender essential oil *or* 3 drops geranium essential oil *or* 1 drop pure rose essential oil (optional). Add the oil to the powder drop by drop, and rub powder between your thumb and forefinger to blend well. Store in a container with a shaker top. Let sit at least overnight before using.

GLYCERIN BATH SOAP

This is a very mild soap that can also be used as a shampoo.

In a bain-marie, place ¼ to ⅓ cup (50-75 mL) grated glycerin soap. Add a pinch of borax. Slowly add 2 cups (500 mL) distilled water or infusion of camomile, rose petals, lavender or chickweed. For infusion instructions, see page 39. Stir until the water is thoroughly incorporated with the soap. When the shampoo has cooled, bottle and label. Let stand for a few days be-fore using.

CHILDREN'S AROMATHERAPY SHAMPOO

In a bain-marie, place ¼ to ⅓ cup (50-75 mL) grated glycerin soap. Add a pinch of borax. Slowly add 1½ cups (375 mL) distilled water and ½ cup (125 mL) aloe vera gel. Stir constantly until the water is incorporated with the soap. When the shampoo has cooled, place a spoonful or two in a small bowl, and mix in 10 drops lavender essential oil and 3 drops petit-grain essential oil. Blend back into the shampoo, bottle and label. Let stand for a few days before using.

HAIR RINSE

To remove any residual soap film from your child's hair after shampooing, rinse hair with a mixture of one part vinegar and eight parts water. Then rinse hair thoroughly with warm water.

CRADLE-CAP TREATMENT

A condition characterized by the formation of a yellowish crust on the scalp of newborns, cradle cap is harmless and usually disappears as the baby's sebaceous glands adjust to life outside the womb. Its primary effect is itchiness. To treat, gently rub into the child's scalp a very thin layer of a mild vegetable oil such as grape-seed, peanut, apricot kernel, rice bran or sunflower. A few drops of calendula infused oil added to the vegetable oil will help soothe any redness or irritation. Leave for a few hours, then wash off with a mild shampoo. (Rub on a few drops of undiluted shampoo first to emulsify with the oil, then add water, and shampoo as usual.) A lot of the crust should rinse off, but don't pick at any remaining bits. This treatment, given no more than once a week, will help control the condition. You can also use the same method for a similar buildup behind the ears.

CHILDREN'S HERBAL BATH

A herbal bath is a gentle treatment for mild skin complaints and a perfect cleansing alternative if a child has exhibited a sensitivity to soap. Make a mild tea using a small handful of one of or a combination of the following herbs, all of which are safe for children: alfalfa, chickweed, marshmallow root, oat straw, red clover, rose petals, sweet clover or sweet violet. Strain, and add to the bathwater.

See also the recipes for oatmeal baths in the chapter "The Bath."

TREATMENTS FOR SUNBURN AND OTHER SKIN CRISES

While caregivers should at all times be vigilant about the extent to which a child's skin is exposed to the elements,

Red Clover
Trifolium pratense

sunburn, windburn, chafing and other redness of the skin seem to be an unavoidable part of growing up. A gentle remedy that can be used on children is the Skin-Saviour Gel described in the chapter "Body Care." If you don't have any on hand, here are some alternative strategies that are also effective for adults.

Aloe Vera Gel: Use purchased gel, or remove a leaf from an aloe vera plant, and squeeze out the gel. Apply a thin layer directly to the affected area.

Cider Vinegar: Apply a cool compress saturated with straight vinegar to the affected area. Replace every few minutes.

Comfrey and Marshmallow: Apply a cool poultice of macerated fresh comfrey root or marshmallow root or a paste made from their dried powder to the affected area. (To make a paste, simply add cold water to the powder.) Replace every 10 minutes or so.

Lavender and Basil: Make a wash (see page 39) of lavender flowers or basil sprigs, or add 10 drops lavender essential oil *or* 2 drops basil essential oil to ½ cup (125 mL) water, and shake. Lightly rinse affected area. Repeat every 2 hours or so, or as necessary.

Potato: Grate some raw potato, or cut in paper-thin slices. Lay on affected area for 10 to 15 minutes. Repeat if necessary.

Yogurt: Apply plain yogurt directly to the affected area, leave on for 5 to 10 minutes, then rinse off. Repeat if necessary. Milk can be substituted.

EARACHE REMEDY

By placing its container in warm water, slightly warm olive oil or an infused oil of mullein flowers or camomile. Test on your wrist before using. The oil should be just slightly warmer than skin temperature. Place several drops in the child's ear, and stop the opening with cotton batting. Leave for a few hours, keeping the child warm, not hot, and protected from drafts. If the earache persists for more than a day, consult a physician.

GLOSSARY

To help demystify some of the language specific to skin care and to the creation of skin-care products, here is a somewhat arbitrary glossary of terms.

ANALGESIC
A compound that eliminates or diminishes pain.

ANTIOXIDANT
A substance that inhibits the rancidity of oils, fats and other materials when exposed to oxygen; common antioxidants are citric acid, vitamin E, beta carotene and ascorbic acid.

ANTISEPTIC
Preventing or counteracting putrefaction, as in wounds; destroys and prohibits the development of microbes.

AROMATHERAPY
The use of essential oils (see the chapter "Ingredients") in the treatment of cosmetic, psychological or medical problems; is a recognized form of medical treatment in France.

AROMATIC
Pleasantly pungent; having a characteristic aroma or fragrance; one of the functions of an aromatic herb is the stimulation of the skin and the olfactory system.

ASTRINGENT
Tending to contract or draw together organic tissues; binding, styptic; in skin care, a substance that causes a minor contraction of the skin, which tightens the pores.

CARRIER OIL

An oil that is used to "carry" other oils, such as infused oils or essential oils that require dilution before they can be applied to the skin. Common carrier oils are sweet almond, olive, sunflower, peanut and apricot kernel.

CONJUNCTIVITIS

Inflammation of the mucous covering of the eyeball.

DEMULCENT

A substance that soothes, especially irritated mucous membranes.

DISTILLATION

The process of heating liquids until they vaporize, then collecting the condensation (see "Essential Oils" in the chapter "Ingredients").

DIURETIC

Tending to increase the flow of urine; enhances the ability of the blood vessels surrounding the ends of the urinary tract to filter out impurities and fluids and increases levels of potassium, sodium and chlorine in the urine.

EMOLLIENT

Having a softening and soothing effect, especially to the skin.

EPIDERMIS

The outer exposed layer of the skin.

ESSENTIAL OIL

The aromatic volatile oil contained in many herbs, flowers and trees. Most are steam-distilled, while some, such as citrus essential oils, are expressed. In varying degrees, they are antiseptic, germicidal and preservative.

EXCRETION

The discharge of waste products from the body, not only through urination and bowel evacuation but also through the sebaceous glands. In fact, the skin is our largest organ, responsible for one-third of our bodily excretions.

GINGIVITIS

Inflammation of the gums.

HUMECTANT

An agent that helps retain moisture in creams and lotions and therefore the skin; two common humectants are glycerin and honey.

HYDROTHERAPY

The treatment of diseases by the external application of water in various forms, such as baths, steam baths and friction rubs.

INFUSED OIL

An oil, usually olive, that through heating and cooling is infused with a plant's beneficial properties. The infused oil can then be used in massage oils, ointments and creams and for general skin care. Calendula, St.-John's-wort, arnica and camomile are all herbs that are typically found in infused oils. Use an inexpensive olive oil as a carrier, because it can be heated and cooled with little change to its molecular structure. Other oils tend to become rancid after the process.

INFUSION

An infusion is basically a tea that is made by pouring boiling water over a herb. The water helps to release the herb's active ingredients. Some barks and berries need to be simmered, covered, for a few minutes, and then left to steep, a method known as "decoction."

MASK

A cosmetic mask is smoothed onto your skin to achieve a particular effect. A clay mask draws oils and impurities from the skin. A mask containing oils, egg yolk and emollient herbs adds moisture to dry skin.

MUCILAGE

A gelatinous substance that contains proteins and chains of chemically linked sugars and has a beneficial action at the point of contact with skin irritations. Plants containing a lot of mucilage are marshmallow, Iceland moss, plantain seed, mullein and comfrey; best processed with as little heat as possible.

ORGANIC ACIDS

These have a mild laxative effect; chief organic acids include malic acid, citric acid, oxalic acid and tartaric acid.

RUBEFACIENT

Any substance that, applied externally, stimulates the circulation; causes warmth and redness, which is useful in treating muscular and rheumatic aches as well as chills.

SAPONINS

A number of natural glycosides that foam in water, making them useful as a gentle detergent; some saponins are toxic if taken internally (see Chickweed and Soapwort in the chapter "Ingredients").

SEBACEOUS GLANDS

Small glands that secrete oily matter to the skin's surface.

TANNIN

Astringent substance related to tannic acid; useful in the external treatment of varicose ulcers, haemorrhoids, minor burns and frostbite; promotes rapid healing and new-tissue formation on wounds and inflamed mucous membranes; for general skin care, it is toning; one of the most common sources of tannic acid is black tea.

TINCTURE

A solution made by soaking a herb in alcohol for a period of time, then straining to remove the spent plant material. This process captures much of a herb's beneficial properties and will keep indefinitely.

TONER

A liquid solution that helps the skin to function. An oily-skin toner is astringent to help draw out oils and tighten large pores; a normal-skin toner is mildly stimulating and emollient; and a dry-skin toner is soothing and emollient.

SOURCES

Finding the ingredients for skin-care products can sometimes be a challenge. Below are listings of Canadian and American businesses that specialize in essential oils, tinctures and herbs.

CANADA

THE AROMATHERAPY SHOPPE
P.O. Box 2605
Bramalea, Ontario L6T 6M5
Phone/Fax 905-451-9375
E-mail: aromashop@aol.com

CHESSWOOD LABORATORIES LTD.
458 Eglinton Avenue W.
Toronto, Ontario M5N 1A5
416-485-0600

HEALTH SERVICE CENTRE
971 Bloor Street W.
Toronto, Ontario M6H 1L7
416-535-9562

THE HERB FARM
323 Parleeville Road, RR 4
Norton, New Brunswick E0G 2N0
506-839-2140

THE HERB WORKS
Unit 5, 180 Southgate Drive
Guelph, Ontario N1G 4P5
519-824-4280; Fax 519-824-2674

THE HERBAL TOUCH
30 Dover Street
P.O. Box 300
Otterville, Ontario N0J 1R0
519-879-6812

KAROOCH ESSENTIAL OILS
Box 2465
Peterborough, Ontario K9J 7Y8
705-749-1894; Fax 705-749-0275

MOLGAARD-WATSON
1325 Rebecca Street
Oakville, Ontario L6L 1Z3
905-847-0266; Fax 905-847-0693

PLANT LIFE
468 Queen Street E.
Box 30
Toronto, Ontario M5A 1T7
416-368-6896
888-690-4820 (toll-free)
Fax 416-368-6896
Also at above address:

WEST WIND SCHOOL
OF AROMATHERAPY
416-368-1426
888-368-1426 (toll-free)

RICHTERS HERBS
357 Highway 47
Goodwood, Ontario L0C 1A0
905-640-6677

UNITED STATES

APHRODISIA
264 Bleeker Street
New York, NY 10014
212-989-6440

ARSENIC AND OLD LACE
318 Harvard Street, #10
Brookline, MA 02146
617-734-2455

BEE CREEK BOTANICALS
Box #204056
Austin, TX 78720
512-331-4244

ENCHANTMENTS, INC.
341 East 9th Street
New York, NY 10003
212-228-4394

FREDERICKSBURG FARM
P.O. Drawer 927
Fredericksburg, TX 78624-0927
830-997-8615

GREENFIELD HERB GARDEN
Box 9
Shipshewana, IN 46565
219-768-7110

HERB PRODUCTS CO.
11012 Magnolia Boulevard
P.O. Box 898
North Hollywood, CA 91603-0898
818-761-0351

THE HERBFARM
32804 Issaquah-Fall City Road
Fall City, WA 98024
206-784-2222

HERBS, ETC.
1345 Cerrillos Road
Sante Fe, NM 87505
505-982-1265

SAN FRANCISCO HERB &
NATURAL FOOD/NATURE'S
HERB COMPANY
1010 46th Street
Emeryville, CA 94608
510-601-0700

THE SOAP OPERA
319 State Street
Madison, WI 53703
608-251-4051 or 800-251-7627
Fax 608-251-1703

WOODSPIRITS LTD., INC.
1920 Apple Road
St. Paris, OH 43072
937-663-4327; Fax 937-663-0100

FURTHER READING

AROMATHERAPY FOR EVERYONE
by Robert Tisserand (Penguin; London; 1988).

AROMATHERAPY FOR WOMEN
by Maggie Tisserand (Thorson's; Wellingborough; 1985).

AROMATHERAPY: THE ENCYCLOPEDIA OF PLANTS AND OIL AND HOW THEY HELP YOU
by Daniele Ryman (Judy Piatkus; London; 1991).

THE ART OF SOAPMAKING
by Merilyn Mohr (Camden House; Camden East; 1979).

THE BOOK OF HOME REMEDIES AND HERBAL CURES
by Carol Bishop (Octopus; London; 1979).

THE BOOK OF MASSAGE
by Lucinda Lidell et al. (Simon and Schuster; New York; 1984).

THE COUNTRYSIDE COOKBOOK
by Gail Duff (Prism Press; Dorchester; 1982).

EVENING PRIMROSE OIL
by Judy Graham (Thorson's; New York; 1984).

THE GARDENER'S BOOK OF HERBS
by Mary Page (Warne; London; 1984).

THE HANDBOOK
OF NATURAL BEAUTY
by Virginia Castleton (Rodale; Emmaus;
1975).
THE HARROWSMITH
ILLUSTRATED BOOK
OF HERBS
by Patrick Lima (Camden House;
Camden East; 1986).
HEALTH FROM
GOD'S GARDEN
by Maria Treben (Healing Arts Press;
Rochester; 1987).
THE HERB BOOK
by John Lust (Bantam; New York; 1976).
HERBAL COSMETICS
by Camilla Hepper (Thorson's; Welling-
borough; 1987).
HERBS FOR USE
AND FOR DELIGHT
edited by Daniel J. Foley (Dover; New
York; 1974).
HOW TO MAKE YOUR
OWN HERBAL COSMETICS
by Liz Sanderson (Keats Publishing;
London; 1979).
MAGIC AND MEDICINE
OF PLANTS
edited by Inge N. Dobelis et al. (Reader's
Digest; Pleasantville; 1986).
A MODERN HERBAL
by Mrs. M. Grieve (Penguin; Harmonds-
worth; 1984).
MODERN HERBAL
by Jeanne Rose (Perigee Books; New
York; 1987).
A NATURAL HISTORY
OF THE SENSES
by Diane Ackerman (Vintage Books; New
York; 1991).
NATURE'S PHARMACY
by Christine Stockwell (Arrow Books;
London; 1989).
THE PENGUIN
DICTIONARY OF BOTANY
edited by Elizabeth Tootill et al. (Pen-
guin; London; 1984).
READER'S DIGEST
ENCYCLOPEDIA OF GARDEN
PLANTS AND FLOWERS
edited by Roy Hay et al. (Reader's Digest;
London; 1978).
THE SCENTED GARDEN
by David Squire (Salamander; Emmaus;
1989).
STAYING HEALTHY
WITH THE SEASONS
by Elson M. Haas (Celestial Arts;
Berkeley; 1981).
THE WOMAN'S BOOK
OF NATURAL BEAUTY
by Anita Guyton (Thorson's; Wellingbor-
ough; 1984).

INDEX